Evidence-Informed Nursing

This introductory text provides nurses with a clear idea of why they should use research information as a basis for high-quality patient care and how they should use that information in the clinical setting. In a logical progression which helps the student build knowledge systematically, *Evidence-Informed Nursing* looks at:

- the rationale for evidence-informed care;
- what research is and approaches to it;
- the benefits of research to clinical practice;
- critical appraisal skills;
- reflective practice and decision-making;
- how to put research into practice;
- the importance of research dissemination.

A summary of essential points to remember is included at the end of each chapter and the text is firmly grounded in the clinical context. It is suitable for use at all levels of training and practice.

Robert McSherry is Principal Lecturer in Practice Development, the University of Teesside. **Maxine Simmons** is Associate Nursing Director, Barnsley District General Hospital. **Pamela Abbott** is Pro-Vice Chancellor, Glasgow Caledonian University.

Evidence-Informed Nursing

A Guide for Clinical Nurses

Edited by Robert McSherry,
Maxine Simmons and
Pamela Abbott

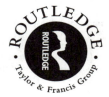

London and New York

First published 2002
by Routledge
11 New Fetter Lane, London EC4P 4EE

Simultaneously published in the USA and Canada
by Routledge
29 West 35th Street, New York, NY 10001

Reprinted 2002

Routledge is an imprint of the Taylor & Francis Group

© 2002 Selection and editorial matter, Robert McSherry, Maxine
Simmons and Pamela Abbott; individual chapters, the contributors

Typeset in Times by M Rules
Printed and bound in Great Britain by
TJ International Ltd, Padstow, Cornwall

British Library Cataloguing in Publication Data
A catalogue record for this book is available from the British Library

Library of Congress Cataloging in Publication Data
Evidence-informed nursing: a guide for clinical nurses edited by
Robert McSherry, Maxine Simmons, and Pamela Abbott
    p. cm.
includes bibliographical references and index
    1. Nursing. 2. Evidence-based medicine. I. McSherry, Robert.
II. Simmons, Maxine. III. Abbott, Pamela.
[DNLM: 1. Nursing Research–methods. 2. Evidence-Based
Medicine. 3. Nursing Care. WY 20.5 E935 2001]
    610.73–dc21   2001019971

ISBN 0–415–20497–6 (hbk)
ISBN 0–415–20498–4 (pbk)

To my wife and children. Thank you Clare for your patience and allowing me endless hours to research this piece of work.

Rob McSherry

To my mum and dad for their lifelong belief in me and to my husband Andrew and children Callum and Georgia for their love.

Maxine Simmons

Contents

Illustrations

Boxes

Figures

Tables

Notes on contributors

Pamela Abbott is Pro-Vice Chancellor at the Glasgow Caledonian University.

Louise Brereton is Lecturer in Nursing Studies at the University of Sheffield.

Jane Haddock is Practice Development Adviser, Surgical Specialities, Chesterfield and North Derbyshire Royal Hospital NHS Trust.

Andrew F. Long is Professor in Health Research at the University of Salford, Manchester.

Robert McSherry is Principal Lecturer in Practice Development at the University of Teesside, Middlesbrough.

Paddy Pearce is Clinical Governance Manager at Friarage Hospital, Northallerton.

Maxine Simmons is Associate Nursing Director, Barnsley District General Hospital.

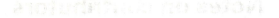

Foreword

Some challenges in doing evidence-based practice

Andrew F. Long, BA (Hons), MPhil, MSc
Professor and Director of the Health Care Practice R&D Unit, University of Salford

With an academic background in sociology, research methods and statistics, Professor Andrew Long has extensive teaching experience at the postgraduate level on health research methods (quantitative and qualitative), the critical appraisal of research evidence and outcome measurement. From 1992–1996 he was Project Leader of the UK Clearing House on Health Outcomes at the University of Leeds, playing a leading role in exploring ways to measure and monitor outcomes within routine clinical practice. Over the past five years, his research has centred in systematic reviews of research evidence on the effectiveness and outcomes of health and social care interventions, and explorations of the role of the nurse within the rehabilitative team, along with continued methodological work in the field of outcome measurement in both complementary and conventional medicine.

In October 2000 the Chief Nursing Officer, Sarah Mullally, and the Director of R&D, Professor Sir John Pattison, widely distributed a paper outlining proposals for action for nursing R&D (Department of Health 2000). Its aim was to explore the best way to achieve the R&D commitments outlined in the nursing strategy document (Department of Health 1999). Central issues addressed include the need to enhance the knowledge, skills and confidence of nurses to do health services research and to use the results of research to support professional practice.

What are appropriate expectations for a practising nurse in this area? There can be little question that every practitioner has an ethical and professional responsibility to ensure that his or her practice is informed by best evidence. This evidence base includes high quality and appropriate research. There is thus a moral imperative on the practitioner to keep up-to-date with research. Reading journals is a first step, moving on to the critical appraisal of relevant articles ('is the study a good one? Is there anything here worth taking up into my practice?'), perhaps participation in journal clubs, and then to integrate the indicated intervention into practice. The key message is to locate, appraise and *use* the research evidence tailoring it to the individual patient.

The onus does not, however, just lie on the practitioner. This requirement must extend to the clinical manager for a service, not least in relation to their accountability for delivering a quality service. More broadly, there are clear implications for the employing organisation. The organisation, down to the ward or smallest base unit, needs to provide supportive and enabling structures and processes to facilitate evidence-based practice. Thus, there needs to be access to libraries (with on-line searching facilities), dedicated/protected time to locate, read and appraise evidence (it is not reasonable to expect this to be done outside of work time) and, perhaps most challenging, empowerment in the workplace to implement (agreed) changes in practice.

A smaller number of nurses will *do* research themselves, on their own, with other nurses and/or colleagues from other disciplines. Part of their task involves ensuring effective dissemination of their research findings. This should be more than the production of an academic article or report (for colleagues to read, critically appraise, etc.). Workshops with targeted potential users of the research findings are needed, together if possible with facilitated sessions on action implications or the development of change management strategies. Indeed, more funders are recognising and requiring researchers to build in a greater emphasis on the 'Development' aspect of R&D.

For research to inform practice it is not just sufficient that it is done well. It also must address the right questions and real problems faced by practitioners within the complexity of clinical practice. Most importantly, it must measure the right things. Health care, and within this the contribution of nursing, is about providing treatment, support, care and advice to individuals. Research studies must thus measure what is important to the patient, as well as the professional. A breadth in perspective over what counts as a successful outcome is necessary, along with ways to capture the effects of the nurse and others' interventions on the patient's experience of the whole treatment and care.

The four-stage model of evidence-based practice, first espoused within medicine and now universally advocated, is powerful. It is, however, incomplete if users of research findings do not systematically and routinely check whether the expected effects are being achieved in practice (Long and Fairfield 1996). This fifth stage, outcomes monitoring within routine practice, addresses the question of, 'once I change my practice, how will I know if my patients have benefited?' (Brown 1999: 112) If the achieved outcomes are not as good as those expected, the next task is to explore reasons why and modify practice accordingly. Implementing evidence-based practice should be a continuous and spiral process.

Against these challenges, this book provides a practical, problem focused and interactive text to assist the practising clinical nurse in ensuring that their practice is grounded on appropriate research evidence. It draws together both academics with interests in the application of research evidence into practice and practising nurses and nurse educators to present and tackle the challenges of doing evidence-based practice.

However, rather than talking about evidence-based nursing, the editors speak more appropriately of *evidence-informed nursing*. Their emphasis lies on the recognition of the nurse (and, by implication, other practitioners) as a *'critical practitioner'* within the context of (professional) accountability.

This characterisation is not a simple refinement of terminology, but a significant change of emphasis and recognition of the real implications of grounding practice on appropriate evidence. As the editors argue in Chapter 1, the nurse must reflect on the range of available evidence and synthesise these to arrive at a defensible judgement and actions in relation to the needs of the individual patient. Their approach also reinforces the five-stage and cyclical nature of evidence-based practice in general, and evidence-informed nursing in particular, through their discussion of the key stage of evaluation within evidence-informed nursing.

The challenge is *doing* evidence-informed nursing. The approaches outlined in this text provide many useful ideas and ways to take this forward. The benefit will be to all, the nursing profession, the quality of health care and, critically, the patient.

Professor Andrew F. Long, University of Salford
February 2001

References

Brown, S.J. (1999) *Knowledge for Health Care Practice* Philadelphia, WB Saunders Company.

Department of Health (1999) *Making a Difference: Strengthening the Nursing, Midwifery and Health Visiting Contribution to Health and Healthcare* London, Department of Health.

Department of Health (2000) *Towards a Strategy for Nursing Research and Development. Proposals for Action* London, Department of Health (PL/CNO/2000/7).

Long, A.F. and Fairfield, G. (1996) Confusion of levels in monitoring outcomes and/or process, *The Lancet* 347, 1572.

Acknowledgements

Thanks to Carol Suter, Practice Nurse, Dr R.F. Hinchliffe and Partners, Clifton Lane Corner Surgery, Doncaster Road, Rotherham S65 1DU, for the research critique in the Appendix.

Chapter 1

An introduction to evidence-informed nursing

Robert McSherry, Maxine Simmons and Paddy Pearce

What is evidence-informed nursing?

Nurses are responsible for the care they provide for their patient. They have to be active, competent and autonomous in providing this care and be able to justify what they do. It is no longer acceptable for nurses to base care on ritual and tradition – they must be able to justify the decisions they have made about appropriate care and treatment on the basis of a professional expertise which includes using research evidence to inform practice.

This book aims to enhance your understanding of, and to subsequently support you in practising, evidence-informed nursing. We use the term 'evidence-informed nursing' in preference to 'evidence-based nursing' in order to recognise that nurses are critical practitioners. It must be sound and relevant research that informs practice. Nurses need to know and understand how to access and use research and how to incorporate it effectively into their everyday practice. They need to acquire and become competent in the skills of research awareness, critical appraisal, reflective practice and decision-making (McSherry 1997). Evidence-informed nursing is the development of a professional practice in which the nurse does something not just because that is how it has always been done or because that is what she/he was told to do, but because she/he has made '. . . a decision for actions which can be justified from a knowledge base' (Marks-Marrah 1993: 123).

This chapter sets the scene by looking at the rationale behind the use of evidence in nursing and at some key definitions and processes associated with it. The following chapters will systematically help you to develop the skills highlighted here as essential to the practice of evidence-informed nursing.

The main imperative for evidence-informed nursing is to ensure the highest possible level of patient care. At the same time proper use of evidence supports nurses in accounting for what they do. Over the last decade there have been significant changes in the expectations placed on nurses by government, employers and the public, with the aim of improving the quality of patient care and achieving clinical excellence. Nurses are accountable to all these groups of people and also to their professional body. A central argument of this book is that a core element of professional nursing is accountability. We recognise, however, that basing practice on evidence is only one element of accountability. Nurses are employed as experts – they are paid to practise on the basis that what they do is well-judged, appropriate and based on an informed appraisal of alternatives. The objective is defensible practice. Nurses should therefore be *critical practitioners*. Ann Brechin (2000) has indicated that critical practitioners:

> conceptualise practice as an open-minded reflective process, build on a sound skills and knowledge base, but taking account of different perspectives, experiences, assumptions and power relations. Critical practice draws on an awareness of wider ethical dilemmas, strategic issues, policy frameworks and social–political context. It acknowledges that there may be no straight forward and 'right answer . . .'
>
> (Brechin 2000: 11)

and

> critical practitioners must be skilled and knowledgeable and yet open to alternative ideas, frameworks and belief systems, respecting and valuing alternative perspectives
>
> (Brechin 2000: 44)

A knowledge and understanding of the relevant research that supports clinical and other nursing practice is only one element of being a critical practitioner, but it is a fundamental one. Evidence-informed nursing is concerned with providing clinically effective patient care and being able to justify the procedures used, the care plan devised or the services provided by reference to authoritative evidence. It is the making of decisions about the care of individual patients and families, on the basis of the best available evidence. French has suggested that it is:

> the systematic interconnecting of successfully generated evidence with the tacit knowledge of the expert practitioner to achieve a change in a particular practice for the benefit of a well-defined client/patient group.
>
> (French 1999: 74)

In other words, evidence-informed nursing is the integration of professional judgement and research evidence about effectiveness of interventions. It provides a sound and rational basis for the decisions taken about patient care by nurses. It requires 'knowledgeable doers', who have the skills and expertise to implement new procedures and policies and who can supervise others involved in providing care to ensure that they carry out procedures in the most appropriate way. (Not everyone involved in *delivering* patient care needs to have the sort of skills and knowledge referred to here, but they are essential for anyone involved in the *management* of the care.) Evidence-informed nursing is a systematic approach to providing nursing care that requires critical appraisal skills. While research evidence on effectiveness is important, it does not require all nurses to be researchers. What it requires is that all nurses have:

- an understanding of the importance of practice being based on the most appropriate evidence on effectiveness;
- access to and the ability to use research findings;

- the ability to evaluate research;
- the ability to implement research findings in their own practice.

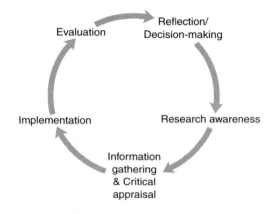

Figure 1.1   The evidence-informed nursing cycle.

Note
Fig. 1.1 demonstrates the cyclical process of how to inform nursing practice with evidence. The process requires reflection on practice, awareness of research, an ability to gather and critically review the evidence, implement the evidence into practice and evaluate the effectiveness of the change in practice. This process subsequently begins again by encouraging the nurse to reflect on the evaluation prompting further decision-making or actions.

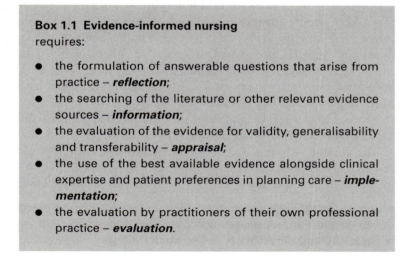

Box 1.1 Evidence-informed nursing
requires:

- the formulation of answerable questions that arise from practice – ***reflection***;
- the searching of the literature or other relevant evidence sources – ***information***;
- the evaluation of the evidence for validity, generalisability and transferability – ***appraisal***;
- the use of the best available evidence alongside clinical expertise and patient preferences in planning care – ***implementation***;
- the evaluation by practitioners of their own professional practice – ***evaluation***.

The move towards evidence-informed nursing is a move away from nursing that rests on a knowledge-base which is unsystematic, towards one where an increasing proportion of nursing decisions are systematic, based on rigorous observation and the testing of treatments and procedures.

How does it relate to clinical effectiveness and evidence-based practice?

Clinical effectiveness and evidence-based practice are increasingly popular terms used in relation to nursing care within a variety of clinical settings. They refer, at least in part, to using research to inform practice and to ensure efficient and effective practice.

The NHS Executive (NHSE) define clinical effectiveness as:

> The extent to which specific clinical interventions when deployed in the field for a particular patient or population do what they are intended to do, that is, maintain and improve health and secure the greatest possible health gain from the available resources.
>
> (NHSE 1996)

Whilst this statement is fairly clear, the emphasis appears to be on what healthcare practitioners will do. The RCN (1996a) definition is more patient-centred, acknowledging the need to consider patient preferences. It refers to clinical effectiveness as: 'applying the best available knowledge, derived from research, clinical expertise and patient preferences, to achieve the optimum processes and outcomes of care for patients' (RCN 1996a).

Reagan (1998) suggests that '. . . clinical effectiveness is the cornerstone of evidence based practice.' However, the RCN (1996b) rather vaguely defined it as: 'doing the right thing in the right way for the right patient at the right time' (RCN 1996b).

Historically, the argument for evidence-based practice developed in medicine. Sackett *et al.* (1997) have defined evidence-based medicine as:

> the conscientious, explicit and judicious use of the current best evidence in making decisions about the care of individual patients. This external information is blended with clinical

expertise in order to decide if and how this evidence may relate to the individual patient. The aim is to inform practice and see if the treatments that are used are the most powerful, accurate, effective and safest options.

However, it is important to note that evidence-based medicine is not the same as research into clinical practice. The latter is based on agendas determined at least in part by researchers themselves. Evidence-based medicine in the UK is based on two things – NHS-determined research needs and the dissemination of findings that are then implemented into practice.

The RCN's definition of clinical effectiveness seems to be very similar to Sackett *et al.*'s (1996) definition of evidence-based medicine. Kitson *et al.* (1997) note that a clearer distinction needs to be made between evidence-based medicine and clinical effectiveness, suggesting that clinical effectiveness has the wider remit of encouraging all staff to question their practice in an attempt to improve patient outcomes. Sackett *et al.*'s (1996) definition of evidence-based medicine values both research evidence and clinical expertise whilst acknowledging the patient's individuality, but not, as in the RCN's definition, patient preferences.

What seems to be missing from all these definitions is recognition of the interdependence of evidence-based medicine and clinical effectiveness; you cannot practise one without the other. Evidence is needed to inform practice; in turn, it is hoped that the improved practice will enhance the patient's experience of a particular intervention, the care they receive or their quality of life, or even all three.

Perhaps this is the rationale for the introduction of the term 'clinical governance':

> a framework through which NHS organisations are accountable for continuously improving the quality of their services and safeguarding high standards of care by creating an environment in which excellence in clinical practice will flourish.
>
> (NHS Executive 1999)

Clinical governance is viewed positively by many health care professionals in that the aim is to improve the quality of life, and health, of the patient (McClarey and Duff 1997). It can be seen as a 'protective mechanism for both the public and health care professionals'

(McSherry and Haddock 1999). Clinical governance requires nurses to practise evidence-based nursing and to have the necessary knowledge, skills and competency to deliver evidence-informed care.

Evidence-based nursing is the 'process of systematically finding, appraising and using contemporaneous research findings as the basis for clinical decisions' (Long and Harrison 1996). Whilst the argument for a move to evidence-based nursing has clearly been influenced by the development of evidence-based medicine and, more recently, evidence-based health care, there are important differences. Evidence-based medicine relies mainly on research using the Randomised Control Trial (RCT) and the systematic analysis of a number of trials in reviews and meta-analyses. Nursing, however, has been committed to developing research using a variety of research methods. There is a dissonance between the core beliefs of nursing and clinical effectiveness. Nurses are committed to providing holistic care (James 1992) as opposed to care based on the biomedical model. Nurses are committed to treat patients as whole people and work with them rather than on them. Furthermore, effectiveness is only one element of the decision-making process – in deciding on the therapeutic intervention others include safety, acceptability, cost-effectiveness and appropriateness (Gray 1997).

Indeed, nurses may value other aspects such as the acceptability to the patient more highly than effectiveness (Robinson 1998). Evidence-based practice takes for granted that the nurse has the right and ability to make the decisions on therapeutic interventions.

It is the case that some elements of nursing, for example wound care, fit easily with the notion of basing practice on evidence, but it is more difficult to relate it to other nursing tasks, such as monitoring, emotional labour, handwashing and other integral aspects of nursing care (Kitson *et al.* 1997). In many cases of nursing work it can be difficult to make firm links between an action and a particular intention. It is often difficult to isolate the nursing intervention from that of other members of the multidisciplinary team and it can be difficult to guarantee measurable and acceptable outcome criteria (Barriball and MacKenzie 1993). Nevertheless, developing nursing practice that is informed by relevant research findings should be an important aspect of nurses' decision-making and, to make this a reality, nurses must understand about research and evidence.

Implementing evidence-informed practice

In this text we prefer to think about evidence-informed nursing – as we have already argued research evidence is only one element, albeit an important one, on which the critical nurse bases therapeutic interventions. In order to achieve evidence-informed nursing a nurse needs to have:

- the research awareness skills and the knowledge and competence to interpret research material and to use it to inform their clinical decision-making;
- a managerial and organisational culture that facilitates the implementation of research into clinical practice.

Evidence-informed nursing is rather more than the practicalities of an individual having to read, interpret and utilise research findings; to be truly effective, it needs facilitation. The correct 'processes' need to be in place to ensure successful implementation, acquisition of the necessary professional skills and reflection on the appropriateness of a given action for a given patient.

To implement evidence-informed practice the individual nurse needs clinical expertise, a knowledge of research evidence, an understanding of patient preferences, adequate resources and an environment that supports the critical practitioner (Figure 1.2) (Cullum, DiCenso and Ciliska 1998).

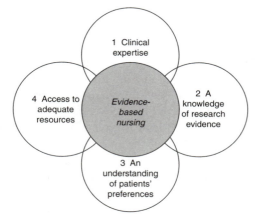

Figure 1.2   Evidence-based nursing.
Source: Adapted from Haynes, R.B. *et al.* (1996).

1 Clinical expertise

Nurses are professionally accountable for the effectiveness of the care they provide (Lo Biondo-Wood and Haver 1990). The United Kingdom Council for Nurses, Midwives and Health Visitors' Code of Professional Conduct (UKCC 1992) makes nurses personally accountable for the care that they provide and imposes on them a duty to monitor and improve their knowledge and competence.

In the last few years, a body of research findings on effectiveness of interventions to underpin professional nursing practice has begun to be developed. Nurses have began to recognise the importance of evidence-informed practice and the need to have the skills to assess the research literature and implement findings in their own day-to-day practice.

2 Knowledge of research evidence

There is increased emphasis on using the latest and highest-quality evidence to inform clinical practice and service delivery, with the aim of improving health outcomes for individuals and the population as a whole. The argument that nursing practice should be research based is not new (see, e.g. Hunt 1981, Garner *et al.* 1976, Roper 1977).

Evidence-informed nursing is a systematic approach to providing nursing care that requires critical appraisal skills. While research evidence is at the center of it, it does not require all nurses to be researchers.

3 An understanding of patient preference and choice

Patients and their families place their trust in nurses. The nurse needs to assess the patient's knowledge and understanding of their condition and involve them in the decision-making process regarding their care. The nurse needs to be able to access and critically appraise the evidence in relation to the care needs of each patient and communicate this information in a style most appropriate to the individual patient.

Patients are no longer passive recipients of nursing care and expect to be involved in and informed about decisions regarding them and their family. Carers do not want to be the passive recipients of professional treatment but to work in partnership with nurses.

(DOH 1999: 9)

4 Access to adequate resources

For nursing to be evidence-informed, research needs to be accessible to nurses who understand the need to base their practice on research and who have the critical appraisal skills necessary to evaluate it, time to access it and skills to implement it (see Chapter 3).

Research evidence may be obtained from the following sources:

- Libraries – text books, journal databases mainly computerised, such as the Cochrane Library that contains systematic reviews; MEDLINE and Cumulative index to nursing and allied health literature (CINHAL).
- Local universities.
- Professional bodies (e.g. Royal College of Nursing (RCN), English National Board (ENB)).
- NHS Centre for Reviews and Dissemination.
- Internet. <www.evidencebasednursing.com> <www.nzgg.org.nz
- Expert opinion.

Strengths of evidence

There are many sources of evidence, so where do you look in the first instance? As a nurse concerned with caring for patients what you need is a guide to the 'best evidence' and where to find it. Muir Gray (1997: 61) provides us with a classification that ranks the evidence (see Table 1.1).

Evidence is categorised according to the overall research studies

Table 1.1 The five strengths of evidence

Class	Strength of evidence
I	Strong evidence from at least one systematic review of multiple well-designed randomised controlled trials
II	Strong evidence from at least one properly designed randomised controlled trial of appropriate size.
III	Evidence from well-designed trials without randomisation, single group pre-post, cohort, time series or matched case-control studies
IV	Evidence from well-designed non-experimental studies from more than one centre or research group
V	Opinions of respected authorities based on clinical evidence, descriptive studies or reports of expert committees

Source: Adapted from Muir Gray (1997).

design in preventing bias from influencing the research findings. For example, McSherry's (1997) study would be categorised as Class III evidence (see Chapter 3). It is worth acknowledging that at this present moment limited Class I evidence is available to underpin nursing interventions. However, the limitation of this hierarchy is that it places scientific or quantitative research studies with higher status than qualitative studies. What needs to be emphasised here is the value of the research in answering the proposed question.

Summary of key points

- No single factor has influenced the development of evidence-based practice.
- Evidence-informed care is about using evidence to support professional decision-making.
- To practise evidence-informed nursing, nurses require knowledge and skills in research awareness, critical appraisal, reflection, decision-making .

Recommended reading

Brechin, A., Browne, H. and Eby, M. (2000) *Critical Practice in Health and Social Care* London, Sage.
Cullum, N., DiCenso, A. and Ciliska, D. (1998) Implementing evidence-based nursing: some misconceptions, *Evidence-Based Nursing* 1, 2, 38–40.
Wilson-Barrnett, J. (1998) Evidence for nursing practice – an overview, *Nursing Times Research* 3, 1, 12–14

References

Barriball, K.L. and MacKenzie, A. (1993). Measuring the impact of nursing interventions in the community setting: A selective review of the literature, *Journal of Advanced Nursing* 18, 3, 401–7.
Brechin, A. (2000) Introducing critical practice. In Brechin, A., Browne, H. and Eby, M. (eds) *Critical Practice in Health and Social Care* London, Sage.
Department of Health (1997) *New NHS: Modern and Dependable* London, HMSO.
Department of Health, (1998) *A First Class Service: Quality in the new NHS* London, HMSO.
Department of Health (1999) *Making a Difference: Strengthening Nursing, Midwifery and Health Visiting Contribution to Health and Healthcare* London, HMSO.
French, P. (1999), The development of evidence-based nursing, *Journal of Advanced Nursing* 29, 172–8.
Gartner, S.R., Black, D. and Phillips, T.P., (1976) Contribution of nursing research to patient care, *Journal of Advanced Nursing* 1, 507–18.
Gray, J.A.M. (1997) *Evidence Based Health Care* Edinburgh, Churchill Livingstone.
Haynes, R.B., Sacket, D.L., Gray, J., Muir, A., Cook, D.J. and Guyatt, G.H. (1996)Transferring evidence from research into practice: The role of clinical care research evidence in clinical decision, *ACP Journal Club* 125, A14.
Hicks, C. and Henesey, D. (1997) The use of a customised training needs analysis tool for nurse practitioner development, *Journal of Advanced Nursing* 26, 2, 389–98.
Hunt, J. (1981) Indicators for nursing practice: the use of research findings, *Journal of Advanced Nursing* 6, 189–94.
James, N. (1992) Care Work and Case Work: A Synthesis? In Robinson, J., Gray, A. and Eltion, R. *Policy Issues in Nursing* Buckingham, Open University Press.

Kitson, A. (1997) Using evidence to demonstrate the value of nursing, *Nursing Standard* 11, 28, 34–9.

Kitson, A., McMahon, A., Rafferty, A. and Scotte, E. (1997) On developing an agenda to influence policy and healthcare research for effective nursing: A description of a national R&D priority setting exercise, *NT Research* 2, 3232–334.

LiBiondo-Wood, G. and Haber, J. (1990) *Nursing Research: Methods Critical Appraisal and Utilization* St Louis, Mosby..

Long, A. and Harrison, S. (1996) Evidence-based decision-making, *Health Service Journal* 106 (January 11), 1–11.

Marks-Marrah, D. (1993) Accountability. In Tschudin, V. (ed.) *Ethics: Nurses and Patients* London, Scutari Press.

McClarey, M. and Duff L. (1997) Clinical effectiveness and evidence-based practice, *Nursing Standard* 11, 52, 33–7.

McSherry, R. (1997) What do registered nurses and midwives feel and know about research, *Journal of Advanced Nursing* 25, 985–98.

McSherry, R. and Haddock, J. (1999) Evidence-based healthcare: Its place within clinical governance, *British Journal of Nursing* 8, 2, 113–17.

McSherry, R. (1999a) Supporting the patient and their family. In Bassett, C.C. and Makin, L. (1999) *Caring for the Seriously Ill Patient* London, Arnold.

Muir Gray, J.A. (1997) *Evidence-based Healthcare How to Make Health Policy and Management Decisions* London, Churchill Livingstone.

Needham, G. (2000) Research in practice: Making a difference. In Gomm, R. and Davies, C. (eds) *Using Evidence in Health and Social Care* London, Sage.

NHS Executive (1996) *Promoting Clinical Effectiveness: A Framework for Action in and through the NHS* London HMSO.

Reagan, J. (1998) Will current clinical effectiveness initiatives encourage and facilitate practitioners to use evidence-based practice for the benefit of their clients? *Journal of Clinical Nursing* 7, 3, 244–50.

Robinson, K. (1998) Evidence-based practice in health building. In Abbott, P. and Weerabeau, L. (eds) *The Sociology of the Caring Professions* London, University College London Press.

Roper, N.C. (1997) Justification and use of research in nursing, *Journal of Advanced Nursing* 2, 365–71.

Royal College of Nursing (1996a) *The Royal College of Nursing Clinical Effectiveness Initiative – A Strategic Framework* London, RCN.

Royal College of Nursing (1996b) *Clinical Effectiveness: The Royal College of Nursing Guide* London, RCN.

Sackett, L.D., Rosenberg, W. and Haynes, B.R. (1996) *Evidence-Based Medicine: How to Practise and Teach EBM* London, Churchill Livingstone.

United Kingdom Central Council for Nursing, Midwifery and Health Visiting (1992) *Code of Professional Conduct* London, UKCC.

Wilson-Barrnett, J. (1998) Evidence for nursing practice – an overview, *NT Research* 3, 1, 12–14.

Chapter 2

Implementing evidence-informed nursing

Research awareness

Pamela Abbott

Introduction

In order to be able to practise evidence-informed nursing an appreciation of what research is, the different approach to research, why we need it and the ethical considerations are essential. The intention of this chapter is to provide the reader with an introduction to these key elements of research awareness. The focus of this chapter is on research methodology to enable nurses to gain an understanding of research to inform their critical reading of it. You may well want to evaluate research findings as a precursor to implementing them in your own professional practice. This may include single research reports that you access. There are now initiatives that enable nurses to gain access to reports that have systematically considered the evidence for clinical interventions. These are of two types – systematic reviews and meta analysis. The former are systematic reviews of all the available research reports on a given clinical intervention that meet the necessary standards for inclusion. If a number of researchers then come to the same conclusion, it increases our confidence that the intervention has a 'real effect'. Meta analysis involves the combining of data from a number of studies that have used exactly the same methods and procedures and then analysing the combined data.

What is research?

The evidence necessary for evidence-based nursing is obtained from systematic and rigorous research. Tradition and 'authenticity', the mainstays of nursing practice in the past, have to be replaced as warrants for practice, where possible, by knowledge from clinical and social nursing research and from research in other relevant social, biological and medical sciences. It is the way in which knowledge is produced and tested that distinguishes research from other ways of knowing (including a problem-solving approach). The Department of Health (1993: 6) suggests that:

> We use the term 'research' to mean rigorous and systematic enquiry conducted on a scale and using methods commensurate with the issues investigated and designed to lead to generalisable contributions to knowledge.

Nursing research is the systematic investigation of nursing practice and the effects of this practice on patient care on individual, family or community health. It is new knowledge generated by finding valid answers to questions that have been raised with respect to the care of patients generally or of a particular group of patients/ clients. The expectation is that research findings will be generalisable beyond the immediate context.

There are a number of types of research: applied work concerned with an immediate problem; evaluation concerned with testing an intervention; and basic work concerned with generating new knowledge or facts, and developing fundamental theories that are not always immediately applicable. Most nursing research is applied – concerned with immediate problems – and much of it involves evaluation of treatments or interventions.

All research knowledge is provisional and open to refutation by further evidence. Research has to be evaluated, not just accepted. Trying to find contradictory evidence is one way of subjecting ideas to challenge. Other key questions are:

- Can the research finding be reproduced?
- Can they be corroborated?
- Can they be applied in other situations?

Beyond looking for contradicting evidence, and evidence that supports the findings, research is subject to technical questions about its *validity* – the extent to which the design of the study and the means of data collection are adequate to produce conclusions which can be declared true beyond reasonable doubt.

In order to evaluate research, then, it is necessary to understand the procedures for undertaking research. However, it is also necessary to recognise that research is more than a set of procedures and techniques for collecting facts. Facts do not speak for themselves, but have to be interpreted and explained. The ways in which research questions are framed and research carried out are also not neutral processes. Research is informed by theory and conceptual frameworks, and research informs and encourages the further development of theory. Theory is the framework within which we make sense of what is going on. Theories assist us both with respect to the decisions about undertaking research and the implementation of research findings. Nursing is informed by a range of theories, including nursing theory.

> Scientific work depends on a mixture of boldly innovative thought and the careful matching of evidence to support or discount hypothesis and theories. Information and insight accumulated through scientific study and debate are always, to some degree, tentative – open to being revised or even completely discarded in the light of new evidence or arguments.
>
> (Giddens 1989: 21)

There have been innumerable debates in nursing about what the appropriate research designs and methods are for carrying out nursing research (see, e.g., the *Journal of Advanced Nursing* over the past ten years). In particular there has been concern that quantitative methods treat patients as objects to be worked on rather than people to be worked with. However, it is now generally recognised that the test of methods is that they should be appropriate to the questions being asked. Nursing research uses a range of methods from the social, biological and medical sciences, including randomised controlled trials, experiments, surveys, in-depth interviewing and participant observation. The research methods that are used should be those that are the best suited for answering the questions which the researcher has designed the study to answer. For example, in order to demonstrate causation it is necessary to carry out a properly controlled experiment; if the intention is to determine whether a new treatment is more likely to benefit patients than existing treatments, then we need to test this by a randomised control trial. What this does not tell us, however, is how patients *feel* about the treatment and what difference it makes to their lives. We may want to know, for example, whether patients find it acceptable to have to take medication. It would be possible not only to carry out the randomised control trial, but also to talk to patients (i.e., hold in-depth interviews with them), to involve carers where appropriate and others who have a stake in the procedure, and to consider the impact that the treatment has on their lives and how they feel about it. This combining of methods is known as *triangulation*.

Why do we need research?

Research is about generating new knowledge and testing existing knowledge, and is essential for improving the standards and quality of patient care. Research carried out by scientists generates knowledge more systematically and rigorously than non-scientists who are simply going about the business of everyday life. The pressure facing many nurses is to develop skills, knowledge and competencies to be able to practise nursing as a 'scientific-based' profession.

Since the publication of the 'Briggs Report' (1977), which stated that 'nursing should become a research-based profession', it appears that nurses have been overcome by a surge in the desire to increase their understanding and utilisation of research. The availability of articles and material seems to be endless, demonstrating a 'proliferation' of activity to justify the need for a 'research-based approach to practice' and the instigation of 'evidence-based care'.

Keteflan (1975), Buckenham and McGrath (1983) and Chandler (1988) support the notion that 'nursing research' is the pathway through which 'professionalism' can be pursued. 'Professionalism' and 'professional effectiveness' may be achieved when 'individuals have learned to maximise their knowledge and skills and are in a 'learning and practice' environment that also maximises the use of their ability' (Deane and Campbell 1985). Deane and Campbell's work surrounding nursing research and the achievement of professionalism seems to be a positive finding and supports the need for research.

The UKCC 'Code of Conduct' (1992) states that 'each trained member is meant to assume responsibility for his/her own continual education and development of practice'. Clark and Hockey's (1979) evidence seems to support the UKCC statement by suggesting that nurses can use relevant research findings, if such findings are available; and the impression obtained from current research literature, such as LoBiondo-Wood and Haber (1990), is that such findings are available and provide indicators for practice. Therefore, it is essential for nurses to utilise the available evidence to practise effective, accountable nursing.

Approaches to research

The first consideration in planning research should be 'is the research necessary?' Research is only necessary if new knowledge or evidence is needed. If rigorous research has already been carried out to answer the questions, then it may not be necessary to carry out further research. The key objective of research is to provide *new* knowledge, although this may include the replication of existing knowledge in different situations, or with different client groups. (While the monitoring of practice is essential, and involves research skills, it is not the same as formal research.) It is also important at this stage to determine that it is ethically possible to carry out the research – that is, that the benefits of carrying out the research outweigh any disadvantages or potential discomfort or harm to patients. Ethical issues are of immense importance for researchers and practising nurses to consider when undertaking or reviewing research as the following section describes.

Ethical considerations in nursing research

Considering the increasing proliferation in the quantity of nursing research, it is imperative that the subjects and researchers have their rights as humans protected. The overriding ethical principle is the concept of non-maleficence where 'those involved in the research come to no harm' (Wagstaff 1998: 34). Clinical nurses have a code of professional conduct to promote ethical practice, and the Royal College of Nursing (1993) has spelt out clearly and in detail the issues relating to nursing research in their document 'Ethics Related to Research in Nursing' which offers a guide to promoting ethical research in nursing.

Ethical considerations for the researcher involve their maintenance of their personal integrity. That is, to accurately and honestly design, implement and report the study findings. The researcher is required to maintain the subjects' confidentiality, anonymity and privacy throughout the entirety of the research. Subjects involved in research should be informed and their consent obtained prior to commencement of the research study. It is important to be aware of the role of the Research Ethics Committees in protecting the subjects from any unethical research practices. When reviewing evidence, the readers need to assure themselves that the evidence was obtained without detriment to the subjects and that they consider the ethical implications of the research findings to their specific clinical area.

This brief introduction into the ethical issues associated with nursing research can be followed up by discussion with your Local Research Ethics Committee and by reading the following recommended works:

Further reading: Ethical issues in research

Cormack, D.F.S. (1996) *The Research Process in Nursing* Oxford, Blackwell Science.
Hammick, M. (1996) *Managing the Ethical Process in Research* Salisbury, Quay Books.
Wagstaff, P. and Gould, D. (1998) Research in the clinical area: The ethical Issues, *Nursing Standard* 12, 28, 33–6.
Royal College of Nursing (1993) *Ethics Related to Research in Nursing* London, RCN.

The stages of a research project

The research needs to be framed so that the researcher's beliefs and initial ideas can be falsified – that is, that they are open to refutation. It needs to start with questions or problems, and proceed to answers based on the interpretation of evidence that can be shown to be valid for the purpose (see Box 2.1). Nurses may be involved in research in a number of different ways: they may participate in/co-operate with research projects, suggest clinical problems for research, use the findings of research in their own professional practice and undertake research themselves.

Experimentation

If the research is intended to test the efficacy of a new drug or treatment, then the research design of preference is the *experiment* – in medicine also described as the *randomised control trial*. This is often held up as the gold standard in terms of research; anything else being seen as second rate and less valid and reliable. However, it answers only some types of questions and indicates only that one type of treatment/intervention is significantly better than no treatment or another type of treatment/intervention. The controlled trial tests the efficacy of a drug or treatment by applying the treatment to one group of people and withholding it from another. To the extent that the first group are exactly like the second in terms of personal characteristics and histories, and that

Box 2.1 The stages of a research project

1   Identifying the problem;
2   defining the questions or problems to be researched;
3   determining what kind of answers will be acceptable;
4   determining what kinds of evidence are needed;
5   collecting essential background information, including a review of the existing literature to determine the theoretical and empirical information that informs the research to be undertaken;
6   the stating of hypotheses or the refined problems to be researched;
7   determining what methods are to be used, that is, how the evidence is to be collected;
8   determining what the sample is to be and how the sample is to be obtained;
9   writing the research proposal and obtaining ethical approval;
10 collecting the evidence;
11 analysing the data;
12 interpreting the findings;
13 reporting the findings;
14 implementing findings in professional practice;
15 monitoring and evaluation;
16 further research as necessary.

they receive exactly the same treatment in all ways except the intervention is administered to the experimental group and withheld from the controlled group, then, logically, any difference between the two which is present at the end, but which is not present at the start, must be due to the administration of the treatment.

The four essential characteristics of the randomised control trial are:

a   a clearly defined treatment;
b   a clearly defined outcome;

c   a comparison of outcome between treatment and non-treatment group or between groups having received different treatments;
d   control of anything else which might have otherwise have explained the observed differences in outcome.

Whilst the control trial is most often associated with drug trials, it is generally the most appropriate method for evaluating a treatment or intervention. It is the only method that permits the establishment of causation. That is, it enables us to say that **a** *causes* **b**, because **a** (the treatment) is the only element of their history that could be responsible for the current difference (**b**) between two previously identical groups. Other methods enable us to say, for example, that **a** and **b** vary together, or even that **a** usually comes before **b**, but they do not enable us to establish beyond doubt that **a** causes **b**. It is difficult to conduct control trials outside of the laboratory, however, and that is where much nursing research is carried out.

Outside the laboratory it is difficult to ensure that the two groups have exactly the same experiences apart from the intervention whilst the control trial is being conducted. That is, it is difficult to guarantee similarity of the experience of the two groups. It is also difficult to ensure that the two groups are identical, or as near identical as possible. There are two methods of establishing an experimental and a control group. The first method is random allocation; that is, patients are randomly allocated to either the experimental or the control group. The second is matched pairs; that is, a number of characteristics that are thought to be important are determined in advance and then patients are matched on these characteristics and one is allocated to the control group and one to the experimental group. The former stands the best chance of 'randomising out' differences, but the two groups need to be quite large. The latter, matching, is difficult to carry out and can control only characteristics that the researcher has thought to include; there could still be substantial unmeasured and unexpected differences.

Whichever method of allocation is used, a further important point about the conduct of experiments/randomised control trials is the ethical considerations that surround having an untreated group; some people are deliberately denied the potentially beneficial treatment for the sake of the research, and many researchers would regard this an unacceptable. A possible compromise is to have one group undergo the new intervention and let the control group be treated with the previously best-available intervention. Another potential difficulty is what is known as the Hawthorn effect (a form of reactivity) – the way subjects respond to the fact that they know they are taking part in an experiment. If the subjects know that they are receiving a new treatment, they may be conditioned by this knowledge as much as by the treatment itself. Even the experimenter is vulnerable to this: knowing that the treatment is experimental may change the experimenter's behaviour in unconscious ways and influence the subjects; the experimenters may behave differently from how they would behave if the treatment was routine. In drug trials it is common to adopt a *double blind* technique so that neither the subjects nor the administering researchers know which is the treatment group and which is the control group. This may be more difficult to establish when the controlled trial is concerned with a new treatment.

For utilisation in evidence-informed nursing, there are a number of potential problems with the use of the experiment/randomised control trial. The experimental design is basically a 'before' measure, an intervention and an 'outcome' measure. The intervention is said to bring about an improvement if the experimental group shows a significant improvement over the control group. However, this does not mean that everyone in the experimental group has benefited from the intervention, nor does it tell us how the subjects *experience* the intervention – whether, for example, the potential benefits outweigh any disadvantage for the patients, or at least some patients. Furthermore, the definition of what is a successful outcome is made by the researcher, not the subjects. The implementation of findings from experiments/randomised controlled trials relies on the professional expertise of the nurse in determining whether the treatment is likely to be beneficial for her patients, in consultation with them. This means not only considering whether the research has demonstrated that the treatment has the desired outcomes, or has better outcomes than other available treatments, but also how that treatment is likely to be experienced by patients. Furthermore, the nurse needs to consider whether the research findings are transferable to her own practice situation.

For example, the research may have been carried out on middle-aged people and may not be equally applicable to older people. The treatment may require compliance with a difficult regime, and the patients may not be willing and able to comply.

Where it is not possible, or it is considered ethically unacceptable to carry out a controlled experiment, it is common to use an 'uncontrolled trial'. In this case the new treatment is introduced and the researcher monitors and evaluates what happens. To obtain interpretable results, careful measurement and exhaustive documentation are essential. It is necessary to have:

a   a measure of the situation before the intervention;
b   a clear and reliable measure or description of what the treatment procedures or programme of change is, so that we know what it is that is causing any change that may occur;
c   a clearly defined set of outcome measures so that we can see what change is brought about;
d   a measurement of anything in the environment that may offer an alternative explanation for the results.

Measurement of the treatment outcome alone is not sufficient. The significance of what the researcher is trying to achieve needs to be clearly stated, as well as what is to count as a successful outcome. However well carried out, this type of research, often referred to as *action research*, is rarely able to establish the efficacy of a treatment or intervention beyond reasonable doubt. Nevertheless, if it is the only possible method, then it gives evidence of a sort – some sort of guide to whether the treatment intervention improves on previous practice.

It may not always be possible to have a randomised control trial with the random allocation of subjects to experimental and control group or the matched pairing of subjects to groups, but it may be possible to carry out a quasi-experiment or a natural experiment. In this situation, the researcher is able to compare two groups, one of which is given the treatment, and one of which was not going to have access to or receive the intervention in any case. In research of this type it is important to ensure that the two groups are as alike as possible in order to be able to say something meaningful about the outcome of the research. For example, research that I was involved in to determine whether it was possible to improve the skills mix in community care collected data in selected areas in Cornwall, one where the intervention was to be carried out and one which was to continue to have the existing skills mix. (It was only after the research was under way that we discovered that one of the two areas used nursing auxiliaries and the other did not. Obviously, this meant that the existing skills mix in the two areas in terms of the delivery of community care was not the same, and it was therefore difficult to determine the impact of the attempts to rationalise the skills mix in the experimental area.) Quasi-experimental comparison is fraught with problems of interpretation precisely because the researcher is generally not in control of what is going on during the experimental period.

Any research designed to test the efficacy of a new treatment experimentally is sought with difficulty because of the difficulty of controlling confounding factors. Patients are people and can make their own decisions and will decide how to behave. Without total control over patients the researcher cannot ensure that, for example, medication is taken at the exact times indicated, that the exercises are done exactly as prescribed, and so on. If more than one person is administering a treatment, they may not do it in *exactly* the same way. Nevertheless, it is essential that new drugs and treatments be tested rigorously, so that it can be demonstrated that potential benefits outweigh potential disadvantages. When a randomised controlled trial is not practical and/or ethically admissible, then other methods that use the logic of the experiment must be utilised, but with some loss of rigour.

Survey research

A survey may be undertaken to answer a number of types of question:

- What is going on?
- Why is it going on?
- What are the attitudes of a client group?

For example, a health authority may be concerned about the number of accidents that older people are having at home. They may also believe that not all accidents are recorded – perhaps only the more serious ones. To implement policies to reduce the number of accidents they may undertake a survey to determine:

a   the number of accidents that older people in their area have had in the last year;
b   the circumstances under which the accidents occurred;
c   the attitudes of older people to the risk of accidents in the home;
d   the risk-taking behaviour of older people; and
e   the groups of older people most at risk – most likely to have accidents (e.g., by gender, age, type of housing).

Surveys may also be undertaken to determine the use of and the attitude towards a service or treatment by a client group – for example, do older people prefer to visit the clinic or have home visits from a practice nurse, and what are the reasons for their preference? Two groups of clients might then be compared, for example, to assess whether the preferences of older people living in rural areas are different from those of older people in urban areas, whether working-class older people have different views from other social groups, etc. Surveys are a sort of case-control study of social needs, trying to predict outcomes or looking for causal links (e.g., whether some forms of nursing care are more effective than others with regard to achieving desired ends, or whether clients who make repeated use of the health visiting clinics differ systematically from those who come once and then drop out). It is not possible to use a survey to establish *causation*, but a survey can establish *correlation* – that is, that two things systematically vary together – and to infer causation because one event precedes the other. A well-known example here is the research into the links between cigarette smoking and cancer. Over the last 30–40 years, research has consistently demonstrated that there is a correlation between cigarette smoking and the development of lung cancer. It is also the case that the cigarette smoking precedes the lung cancer, and it can therefore be inferred that cigarette smoking is responsible for the development of lung cancer. However, it is not possible to establish causation fully, because it is not possible to establish fully that there is *no* third factor that is responsible both for people smoking and for lung cancer.

The usual stages of a survey's design are:

1 Formulating the problem or area of study, as precisely as possible after reviewing the literature.

2 A pilot stage for talking to potential respondents in fairly open and unstructured ways about the topics of surveys to get their ideas and some notion of the terminology they use.

3 Defining where the research is to be carried out, for example, in a few institutions in one or several wards, etc.

4 Selecting the sample of respondents, or settings, or devising rules for how a sample is to be picked.

5 Deciding on the best mode of delivery. Whether you are going to observe behaviour in a systematic way or ask questions. If you decide on a questionnaire, would it be administered by an interviewer, sent by post for self-completion, or delivered by some other means? At the same time, you would plan what to do about refusals and non-response, whether to send follow-up letters and whether it is possible to collect any descriptive information about people who refuse to co-operate.

6 Thinking carefully about what descriptive demographic information might be necessary or useful; age, gender, social class, etc., and precisely how to record it.

7 Thinking what alternative explanations might be offered for any results obtained and what extra information needs to be collected to explore them ('third factors' as discussed above).

8 Designing the questionnaire or observation schedule. If this includes measurement scales not in common use, a second stage of pilot work would be needed to check on the validity of the measures. Looking for evidence that they do measure what you want and their reliability, i.e., that they produce fairly stable consistent results. In a final pilot stage, you would try out the questionnaire or schedule to identify and deal with problems in its administration. At this stage, it would also be necessary to think about how results are to be analysed and to ensure that the data will be recorded in a suitable form.

The above stages apply to the cross-sectional survey, designed to determine what the case is at present, and asking a sample of people about it at that time. When looking at changes over time, more sophisticated designs such as longitudinal surveys are required.

The most common form of survey is one that uses questionnaires asking people questions about themselves, what they think and believe. However, surveys do not have to ask people questions. The systematic observation of behaviour is an equally important survey technique and, where it is applicable, it may be a stronger approach than verbal questioning. The researcher does not have the difficulty of interpreting the sense which respondents have made of the questions and what they mean by their answers. As a survey technique, observation must be systematic – it must entail counting or measuring behaviours in some consistently reliable fashion.

The ideal survey is a census, questioning every member of a population – for example, every nurse or every patient in a hospital, or every household in an area. This is seldom practical, however, and so researchers have to sample their population. It is important that a sample is representative of the population from which it is drawn if a valid generalisation is to be made. For example, if a health visitor wishes to survey the attitudes of her clients to home visits, it is essential that her sample is representative of all her clients. There are a number of ways of obtaining representative samples. The best kind of sample for survey work is the random sample, one drawn from a complete list of the population – that is, of those to whom we want the results to be generalisable. (In the example above, the health visitor should select randomly from a complete list of her clients.) The sample has to be selected in such a way that every member of it has an equal chance of being represented and it is chance that determines which particular members are selected. (Note that in the example above some older people may not be on the GP's list (e.g. travellers); to the extent that these differ in significant ways from other older people, the findings of the research may not be generalisable to them.)

As a random sample is *random*, drawn by chance, it is reasonably likely to be roughly representative of the population, but only roughly. It is possible to improve the representation by a process know as stratification – separately sampling the strata (layers) of the population using a variable known to be of some importance –

for example, gender and/or age. If you know that gender is an important variable in terms of the research question, you can improve the representative nature of your sample in this respect by drawing separate samples of males and females in numbers proportionate to the numbers of the two in the population.

Frequently, when drawing samples from the world at large rather than a particular institution or setting, a random sample is not possible because there is no list of the population from which to draw it. Alternatively, random sampling may be inappropriate because the spread of a true random sample would be too great for any researcher to handle. A random sample of 500 older people scattered across the British Isles would not give more than one or two in each town, and a national random sample of hospital patients would not be much more accessible. Here, researchers resort to what is known as 'cluster sampling', picking geographical samples and then sampling within them. There is a risk that the sample will be unrepresentative because the range is constricted. However, you can apply the principle of stratification to overcome this risk by selecting your clusters according to some sensible system.

Quota sampling is a procedure which attempts to obtain a representative sample by non-random means. Important variables are defined in advance, the numbers in the population determined, and interviewers then required to interview the numbers of people in each quota, for example, elderly middle-class women, working-class men and so on. This procedure will guarantee that the sample is representative with respect to the variables which are used to form the quotas. However, there is no control over other variables, and quite serious biases can therefore creep into the sampling. Care should be taken in using the results from surveys using quota sampling unless there is additional evidence to support the conclusions.

As the aim of survey research is generalisability, it is important that the sample is representative of the population and that the results are only generalised to that population. (If research is carried out into women's attitudes to a new counselling service, it is not possible to generalise the results to estimate men's attitudes. However, the results of the research may give some guidance as to what research to carry out in order to determine men's attitudes.) The survey can be used to ask a whole range of demographic questions, straightforward questions about behaviour or belief, and can utilise complex scales made up of items known to correlate with some aspect of personality or attitude – that is, personality or attitude scales

Qualitative research

The types of research that I have discussed above – experiments and surveys – are often referred to as *quantitative* research. *Qualitative* research is research that seeks to tell stories. That is not to say that it tells falsehoods or fictions; what it does is to try to make sense of what is going on from the perspective of participants. What is it like, for example, to care for a highly dependent relative? How do pregnant women experience the care they receive from doctors and midwives? We can examine questions such as these only by listening to and helping to recreate people's stories.

Truth is the overall aim of research, whatever its style. If people are not convinced that conclusions about the world are likely to be true, then nothing else about the research will be convincing. It is often argued that qualitative research finds it more difficult to establish the truths of its conclusions than quantitative research, lacking precise measurement and clearly defined concepts. However, neither style finds it easier or more difficult than the other, and qualitative research is quite as rigorous as quantitative research when properly conducted and in circumstances which allow for rigour.

There is a wide diversity of qualitative methods and common issues on which all qualitative research focuses. The practicalities of qualitative research are design and getting into the field, case selection, managing the project, collecting the data, the analysis of data for a variety of purposes and the ethics and politics surrounding the research. In other words, they are precisely the same considerations as those faced by quantitative researchers.

People often tend to talk about qualitative research as if it were one thing with a single set of aims and purposes and techniques. This is a myth, however, and there is a whole range of qualitative methods, intended to provide different types of information. In nursing research, the type of qualitative work most used is what we could refer to as applied qualitative research. A considerable body of qualitative nursing research has now been developed which informs practice in nursing. Qualitative research, for example, on the social conditions of hospitals and particularly psychiatric hospitals (e.g., Goffman 1961, Caudill *et al.* 1952, Rosenhahn 1973) have long formed part of the history of medicine and medical treatment. Qualitative studies of medical and nursing socialisation have also been very influential (Becker *et al.* 1961, Atkinson 1981, Melia 1987, Dingwall 1977). Current scientific medical knowledge, as I have suggested above, places great faith in the randomised control trial and the precise measurement of input and output conditions, and the medical profession often hold up these methods as universally superior to the more qualitative knowledge-base typical of, for example, nursing. To accept this claim, however, would be to deny the insights offered into treatment, decision-making and living with pain which have been offered by a number of important qualitative studies (e.g., Locker 1981, Cornwell 1984). It is also to ignore feminist work on pregnancy and childbirth (e.g., Oakley 1980, 1984), whose impact has effectively revolutionised practice in this branch of the medical profession. Little by little, even medicine is coming to accept that qualitative data has as much of a role to play as quantitative in an applied science.

There are three main qualitative methods used in evidence-informed practice: *participant* (or *qualitative*) *observation, in-depth interviewing* and *focus group* interviewing. Participant observation is the broadest and most naturalistic form and a relatively unstructured form of research: observing in a natural setting as a participant. This is one way in which situations have been explored from the perspective of participants with (ideally) minimal imposition of researchers' or management's preconceived ideas. It is also one of the ways in which a nurse may investigate her own practice in the widest possible way: looking not at how some particular practice works, but at how in general her professional life is conducted, what it means and what the implicit working rules are. Participant observation can also be seen as the most dangerous way in which research can be conducted. It can be destructive of relationships, it can upset and side-track professional practice, and the methodological imagination can sometimes be stretched to the point where the researcher's very sense of identity comes under attack. It is also quite possible for great damage to be done to the people in the context being researched, if the impact of the research is not being constantly monitored.

Classic *participant observation* is where a researcher becomes part of the context without participants knowing that they are a researcher: *covert* (hidden, secret) participant observation. This method of research is now mostly considered to be unethical, although it is still occasionally undertaken. Research has been carried out using this strategy – for example, on young people or unemployed people, deviant sexual groups or religious sects, and indeed in health care settings. It is now more usual, however, for the researcher to explain to the participants that the research is taking place, even though they then become a member of the group. For example, Robert Dingwall studied socialisation into the health visiting role by joining a group of trainee health visitors, but explicitly as a researcher. Indeed, it would have been difficult for him to do otherwise as at the time when he undertook the research, only women were able to train as Health Visitors. However, even when the participants know that they are being researched, they may well forget it, as the researcher becomes an accepted member of the group.

There are a number of problems with participant observation. First, gaining access to groups is not unproblematic. It is, of course, possible for nurse researchers to carry out research in their own places of work, which solves the access problem, but raises ethical ones. Otherwise, it is necessary to join a group, and then there will be gate-keepers with whom negotiations have to be carried out and permissions gained. A second problem is limitation on access or freedom to 'move around the field' – failing to gain access to all situations and so missing important information. In the health visiting research, for example, Dingwall indicated that he may have missed valuable information by not having access to conversations students had in the toilets. The third problem, mundane but crucial, concerns data collection. Even in overt participant observation it is still very unnatural to take notes in many settings, and it can intrude on the normal day-to-day operation of the setting. (Often, however, notes *can* be taken in nursing research, because it is quite common for note-taking to occur on hospital wards and in other sittings where nurses are caring for patients.) Whatever strategy is adopted, it is, of course, necessary for records in participant observation to be as full as possible. Researchers cannot rely fully on memory.

The full-blown participant enquiry is not just an intuitive description; it is about getting a feel for what is going on, or trying to make sense of what is happening in terms of the participants. As the observation progresses, ideas will begin to emerge as to what is important within the context, and the research will progressively pay more attention to some features of the situation than others. This *progressive focusing* is the first stage of theory building, trying to establish what is important or interesting in the situation. As time goes on, the theme will become clearer and a tentative theoretical model of the situation will begin to be put forward. This will be refined and tested by theoretical sampling: testing the generality and the boundaries of an idea by extending the sample of informants or situations systematically and purposively. For example, working in a hospital, a nurse researcher would check that her/his emerging ideas held for the night shift as well as the day nurses, for all types of wards, and for auxiliaries, aids and students as well as for qualified nurses. She/he might then make very specific comparisons – male and female nurses, older nurses and younger ones, theatre nurses and ward nurses – according to what the emerging predictive model suggested. Once a model has been developed, the researchers will then look to falsify and look for cases that were not confirmed.

The major risk with overt participant observation is *reactivity*, the way in which the presence of the researcher and her/his behaviour alters the situation, which might have been quite different if the researcher had not been there. If we take the example of Robert Dingwall's research on health visiting, he was the only male and a researcher. If he had not been in the class, the dynamics and the ways in which the health visitors developed their professional identities may have been very different.

However, the overarching methodological problem with reports based on participant observation data is the problem of validity. Why on earth should anyone take the word of the researcher that what they have claimed to have seen and heard is what any other reasonable person would have extracted from the situation? Research should be illustrated with quotations and extracts from field notes, and those reading and using the research have to trust that the researcher interpreted what they saw, heard and experienced in the same way as others would have done. There are more formal 'guarantors of validity' to which researchers may appeal, however, and the two principle ones are triangulation and reflexivity.

Triangulation, a metaphor drawn from navigation, means taking more than one bearing on a point in order to locate it uniquely. In research terms, it means being able to show that more than one source has been used, each with its own bias, but not necessarily the same bias in each case. Thus, observation is supplemented with interviews to show what the researcher has concluded from observing behaviour is what the participants also understand by it, or at least what the research concluded made sense to the participants. The researcher may draw on important conversations heard in staff rooms, toilets, etc., to supplement formal interviews and may use diaries, letters or articles which participants have written for the newspapers, and so on. In order to extend the range of perspectives, the research may have used more than one observer, perhaps located in different parts of the research field to elicit different viewpoints and different interpretations. Each of these sources leads to an account, and no account is necessarily privileged over other accounts, but to the extent that differently based accounts appear to agree, we may have more faith in the results. To the extent that they do not agree, further research may be needed before it can provide the basis for evidence-informed nursing.

Reflexivity is of even more importance. At every stage of the research, right from the initial introductions, researchers should be thinking about how the participants are making sense of their presence, what they are taking for granted, or learning as new about the subjects and how what they are doing may be shaping a particular piece of data or the whole relationship between them and the participants. Reflexivity is important for three reasons:

1   It acts as a form of self-monitoring so that researchers can spot when something is going wrong and correct it.
2   It is a form of data analysis, one way in which researchers find

their way through the morass of material towards the underlying model, which simplifies and makes sense of what is going on.

3   It is the basis of the researcher's self-justification in the eventual report – a way of showing that others should believe that the researcher's interpretations are reasonable.

Open *in-depth interviewing*, a second prime method, is a naturalistic way of talking to people, making sense of what is going on here by asking participants to let you know. Open interviewing is not one method, but a term for a range of procedures that have:

1   the aim of eliciting the informant's views in the informant's own terms;
2   an attempt to make the interviews resemble natural conversations as far as possible; and
3   the desire to impose as little as possible of the researcher's idea on the conversation.

Those using in-depth interviewing have a wide range of ways of using it. Some interviews are virtually undirected by the researcher, with the informant controlling most of the direction of the conversation, whilst in others the interviewer takes more control, trying to cut through irrelevance and keeping the informants to the point. Most interviewers go in with an outline agenda, but for some this consists only of a list of topic areas to be covered and a few stock questions to get things started and bridge gaps in the conversation. In other cases, however, the researcher may have a more detailed list of questions to ask of all informants and may even try to determine the order in which they are answered. Mostly, we adopt a neutrally sympathetic manner when interviewing, but in some research – for example, on managers of large corporations – the researchers have thought it appropriate to adopt an adversarial style and provoke an argument in order to test the informant's beliefs. All of these are valid ways of doing interview research and each has its strengths and corresponding weaknesses. On the whole, the more structured the approach, the less naturalism and the more danger of attributing the researcher's ideas to the informants. On the other hand, structure makes for uniformity in coverage and so for more interpretable data. At its simplest, the open interview is a way of finding out what people think about a situation, with the minimum of imposed structure necessary to keep the focus of the interview within bounds and avoid having to listen to totally extraneous material. In the less structured open interview, people talk about the situation and what matters to them. This enables the researchers to find out what is salient to them, and what most readily comes to their lips. A more structured approach would be to use an agenda of areas to be covered, so that we can be sure that all informants have covered the same ground. It is necessary, however, to be careful about how such an agenda is used and how the particular topics are introduced, to avoid imposing the researcher's structure on informants and thereby failing to get at what is salient to informants and their views and ideas.

A final method of qualitative research often used in evidence-based nursing is the *focus group*. Focus groups are often used to increase the number of respondents interviewed, and also because they allow interaction to take place. A focus group is an in-depth, open-ended group discussion, usually lasting for one or two hours. Each focus group typically consists of 5–8 participants plus the facilitator(s). Focus groups can be used in the evaluation of the quality of care, for example, to interview people about their perception of a service, to develop ideas for further research, and/or to generate more critical comments than would be available in structured questionnaire-based interviews. They are used because they are more natural and provide an opportunity to find out how informants feel about a situation, to get under the taken-for-granted stock answers. In other words, a focus group methodology is similar to that of an open interview, but with a group of people. The advantages of the focus group methodology over, for example, individual in-depth interviews, are:

1   The amount and range of date is increased when collecting from several people at the same time.
2   There is, to some extent, natural quality control – there are checks and balances, and extreme views tend to be weeded out.
3   Group dynamics often enable important topics to emerge and be challenged, so that it is possible to probe and to uncover what the important topics are for the informants as a group.
4   The method is relatively inexpensive and flexible.

5 It can empower some participants – some people feel more able to talk in a group interview and prefer that method to being interviewed on their own.

6 It enables clarification and cross-clarification between different people to determine that they are talking about the same sorts of things.

7 It is often easier to discuss taboo subjects in focus groups – people tend to be less inhibited in groups and researchers are less inhibited about raising sensitive topics.

There are also a number of disadvantages in focus groups:

1 The number of issues and questions that can be raised is limited – even more limited than in individual in-depth interviews, because there are a number of people.

2 The method requires expertise, probably even more expertise than other research methods. To run a focus group requires two people: a facilitator and someone to take notes and operate the tape recorder.

3 It needs to be facilitated in such a way that all participants are enabled to contribute.

4 Conflicts or power struggles may occur, which need to be managed by the facilitator.

5 People may be reluctant to express certain views or to reveal certain things within a focus group because there are other people there.

6 As with all qualitative methods, there is the problem of generalisability.

Qualitative methods have the advantage, then, that they enable the researcher to ask questions about what is really going on and to understand things in terms of the informants and to get more in-depth answers than if we used questionnaires. Their major drawback is that they can generally involve only a small number of people, the samples are not representative, and therefore generalisability is problematic. However, qualitative work can underpin evidence-informed practice and is an important way of making sense of and understanding people's lives. Qualitative research has been important, for example, in developing policies in the area of community care and in the management of pregnancy and childbirth. In-depth interviewing has, in particular, revealed the burden that informal carers have faced in providing care for heavily dependent relatives.

Conclusions

The vast majority of nurses will never undertake research, although they may participate in research or co-operate with researchers. However, they will need to monitor their own practice, to determine if what they are doing is working well and, if not, to adapt their care plans as necessary. Patient care is individualised care, while research findings are based on statistical significance and/or description of what works for most people. The research-based treatments may not work for all patients, the same pattern of service delivery may not work for all clients, and the preference of the majority is not necessarily the preference of all. There will always be a need for the skilled and experienced practitioner to mediate the conflicting claims of research, to adapt its recommendations to the particular case and to monitor its performance. Increasingly, however, the experienced practitioner will include an understanding of research methods and an *informed* scepticism about research conclusions among her professional skills. Research awareness can only be achieved by having an understanding of what research is, the various approaches to research, why we need research and the ethics of nursing research.

Summary of key points

- Research is systematic and rigorous enquiry, which uses methods appropriate for the issues under investigation.
- We need research to inform nurses of what are the best proven practices.
- Evidence-informed nursing is dependent upon having an understanding of the various approaches to research and the research process. An awareness of the broader issues associated with this aspect of evidence-informed nursing is essential in evaluating the suitability of research for a specific situation.

Recommended reading

Corrim, R. and Davies, C. (2000) (eds) *Using Evidence in Health and Social Care* London, Sage.

Cormack, D.F.S. (1996) *The Research Process in Nursing* Oxford, Blackwell Science.

Polit, F.D. and Hungler, B.P. (1995) *Nursing Research: Principles and Methods* J.B. Philadelphia, Lippincott Company.

Holloway, I. and Wheeler, S. (1996) *Qualitative Research for Nurses* Oxford, Blackwell Sciences.

References

Atkinson, P. (1981) *The Clinical Experience: The Construction and Reconstruction of Medical Reality* Aldershot, Gower.

Becker, H., Hughes, E.C. and Strauss, A.L. (1961) *Boys in White: Student Culture in Medical School* Chicago, University of Chicago Press.

Briggs, A. (1977) *Report of the Committee on Nursing* London, HMSO.

Buckenham, E.J. and McGrath, G. (1983) *The Social Reality of Nursing* Bristol, Health Service Press.

Caudill, W., Redlich, F.C., Gilmore, H. and Brody, E.B. (1952) Social structure and interaction process on a psychiatric ward, *American Journal of Orthopsychiatry* 22, 314–34.

Chandler, V.J. (1988) Science, knowledge and research: What and why for nursing, *Orthopaedic Nursing* 7, 3, 41–4.

Clarke, J. (1994) Moral dilemmas in nursing research, *Nursing Practice* 4: 4, 22–5.

Clark, J. and Hockey, L. (1979) *Research for Nursing: A Guide for the Enquiring Nurse* Aylesbury, HMM.

Cornwell, J. (1984) *Hard-Earned Lives* London, Tavistock.

Deane, D. and Campbell, J. (1985) *Developing Professional Effectiveness in Nursing* Virginia, Rector Publishing Company.

Department of Health (1993) *Report of the Taskforce on the Strategy for Research in Nursing, Midwifery and Health Visiting* London, Department of Health.

Dingwall, R. (1977) *The Social Organisation of Health Visitor Training* London, Croom Helm.

Giddens, A. (1989) *Sociology* Cambridge, Polity Press.

Goffman, E. (1961) *Asylums: Essays on the Social Situation of Mental Patients and Other Inmates* New York, Doubleday Anchor.

Himmelweit, S. (1988) In the Beginning. In Open University Course D211, *Social Problems and Social Welfare* Milton Keynes, Open University.

Keteflan, S. (1975) Application of selected nursing research findings into practice, *Nursing Research* 24, 2, 89–94.

LoBionde-Wood, G. and Haber, J. (1990) *Nursing Research: Methods, Critical Appraisal and Utilization* Toronto, Mosby.

Locker, D. (1981) *Symptoms and Illness* London, Tavistock.

Melia, K. (1987) *Learning and Working* London, Tavistock.

Oakley, A. (1980) *Women Confined: Towards a Sociology of Childbirth* Oxford, Martin Robinson.

Oakley, A. (1984) *The Captured Womb* Oxford, Blackwell.

Royal College of Nursing (1993) *Ethics Related to Research in Nursing* London, RCN.

Rosenhahn, D. (1973) Being sane in insane places, *Science* 179, 250–8.

UKCC (1992) *Code of Conduct* London, UKCC.

Chapter 3

Critically appraising research studies

Andrew F. Long

Introduction

As identified in Chapter 1, there are many reasons for needing to be able to ground nursing in appropriate research evidence. These include rising patient and carer expectations, innovations in medical and information technology and changes in educational provision

Within this chapter, the reader is provided with essential information and the skills to be able to read and appraise both journal articles and research findings in a critical and constructive fashion. This is achieved by providing a systematic framework made up of the essential facts needed to understand, relate and evaluate information relating to the research process. The chapter discusses and examines in detail how the practice of evidence-informed care is associated with an awareness of the key aspects of the research process as illustrated in Box 3.1.

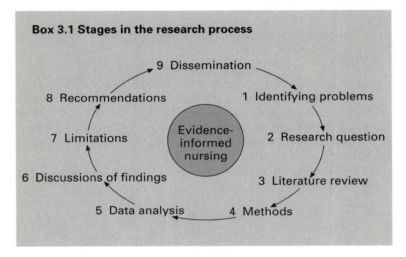

Box 3.1 Stages in the research process

The chapter emphasises the importance of understanding how the research question or practical problem is the catalyst for adopting appropriate research methods and approaches. Finally, Carol Suter provides a critique of an article by McSherry (1997) undertaken as part of her undergraduate studies using a similar approach to the one outlined in this chapter.

So, what information is needed in order to be able to critically appraise a research paper, report or any written information? This chapter will systematically work through the following headings to provide the reader with the essential tools to critically appraise research literature:

- The Context
- What is Critical Appraisal
- Beginning an Appraisal
- Key Criteria for Research Studies
- A Set of Evaluative Appraisal Tools

Case study 3.1

The starting point

As a registered nurse, midwife or health visitor a colleague approaches you and asks one of the following:

- There is an interesting article in the recent copy of the *Journal of Advanced Nursing*. Could we use the approach outlined in the work of the unit?
- During a recent visit to the library, I came across a set of papers arguing for the benefit of the four-layered bandage. The findings seemed powerful to me. At present this is not the way that venous leg ulcers are being treated in the unit. Should we be using this approach in our care delivery?

What should you do? Read on.

Feedback

These snapshots present typical situations where the nurse, or any other health or social care practitioner, will come across research studies in the course of her work. The simple question 'What should you do?', however, has a number of answers. One of these forms the focus and thrust for the content of this chapter. An appropriate reply might be:

- 'Well, it depends. Are you confident that the findings are valid, and thus worthy of being taken up into your nursing practice? Is there anything about the way the study was done that may make you change your mind or deter you from applying the findings in your practice?'

The context

Appraising research evidence has a long history (see, for example, Stern 1975). It has, however, come to be highly fashionable with the upsurge of interest and advocacy of evidence-based practice (or the rather narrower notion of evidence-based medicine) (Rosenberg and Donald 1995, Long and Harrison 1996, Sackett *et al.* 1996a and 1996b). Good research has always built on previous knowledge. Indeed, the aim of research is to extend knowledge and, by implication, to establish best practice – 'what is the right/best thing to do?'

At one time, many questioned the value of the development and use of checklists of methodological questions to assist in appraising research studies. Understandable doubts were raised about the 'messiness of research' and the 'inevitability' of studies being found wanting. In part, these doubts are fair. Doing research never is quite like what is described in the textbook. At the same time, in today's world practice must be evidence-based. This should mean 'grounded in appropriate – research – evidence'. At the same time, it is important to remember that research is only one form of evidence; experience and professional judgement are yet other, important forms.

The ability to appraise research studies has become a *sine qua non* within modern health and social care professional practice. The relevant evidence will, however, include a wide gamut of studies employing different types of research design, qualitative and quantitative, as well as systematic reviews. The 'new' health care worker needs proficiency across methods, if she/he is to make sound judgements about what research findings to take into practice.

To appraise research studies requires an understanding of the nature, principles and key concepts of research as explained in Chapter 2. The focus of this chapter is to build upon previous chapters and to provide the reader with insight into ways to constructively appraise such a range of research studies. It presents a set of evaluative tools. These are based on a systematic framework of key questions about the way a particular study is undertaken. In so doing, the reader will be introduced to key concepts within the research process.

However, reading about critical appraisal is no substitute for 'doing' critical appraisal. Confidence and competence can only be gained by practice. This means dedication – to apply your critical faculties to each research article you read. Seek help from your colleagues. Join a journal club. So, in reading through this chapter, pick up an article and begin to apply the evaluative frameworks to it. Then share your evaluative comments with a colleague. Listen to their comments, reappraise the article, testing and refining your skills and building up your confidence.

What is critical appraisal?

Appraising research is a process of *constructive* review or criticism, aimed at *coming to a judgement* about the value of a piece of research. Is it a 'good' or a 'poor' study? It involves identifying strengths, weaknesses, relevance and action implications for policy and/or practice. By extension, it should also suggest ways that the identified weaknesses could have been addressed in the study under review and/or in future studies. Most importantly, constructive evaluation requires an explanation of *how* and *why* this judgement was arrived at.

Flaws can be found even in the best research report. The critical question is, does this flaw invalidate the findings of the research? Does it provide a tenable counter hypothesis, or alternative explanation, of the findings of the study? To take a simple example, a small sample size should suggest caution in generalising the study's results; it does not make the study's findings invalid. Not controlling for the smoking status of participants in a study where smoking may be a potential cause does. Again, in this light, it is important to review a study *in its own terms*. The authors, rightly or wrongly, may have chosen to use a one-group design when a comparison group was really needed. The appraiser must first judge the quality of the study that was undertaken/reported on, and only later return to the question of the relevance of the particular design to answer the research questions.

Beginning an appraisal

Most of us when reading a journal article will scan through it quickly, noting particular parts of interest or significance. More generally, we may read only the abstract of an article. That may then be the end of the story. Either the study coheres with our previous beliefs or knowledge about the area – we go away reinforced – or it challenges us in some way. A closer look is called for.

Box 3.2 Is an abstract a good guide to a research report?

The initial results of an on-line bibliographic literature search are abstracts, though some databases do not provide abstracts on all included items. Structured abstracts, now required by a number of journals, for example the *British Medical Journal*, make abstracts a closer reflection of the content of an article. But, it is important to remember that an abstract is most commonly a selective indicator of the article. In general, it is there to entice the potential reader to read on. Beware! (See Narine *et al*. 1991, Froom and Froom 1993, Haynes 1993)

Becoming a more critical reader requires a change in approach. We need to interact with the report. Careful and close reading is needed. Prior to deciding on the potential clinical significance or action implication of the findings, we must engage with the way the study was done, the appropriateness of the design and execution of the research study. Each section of the research report is of interest and the likely location of key information to assist in appraising the quality of the article and its relevance for practice (Box 3.3).

Not all studies will provide this information. Sometimes, it may be unclear what the aims of the study actually were; instead, the authors have talked in general terms. Or, it may be only in the results section that it becomes evident what the study is actually studying. In contrast, an indicator of a 'good' study is the authors' commenting critically on their own study within the discussion section of the report. More commonly and problematically, because of the limitations of space in any journal report, detail on methods may be lacking.

Box 3.3 Sections of an article and potential sources of information for appraisal

Introduction	Theoretical and practical rationale for the research. Indications of gaps in knowledge and problems with previous research studies. Aims and hypotheses of the research. Research funder/sponsor.
Methods	Insight into how the study was done, for example: research design, sample, data collection and analysis approaches, and ethical issues.
Findings/Results	Match of the findings to expectations and study aims. Data analysis in practice.
Discussion	Interpretation of the findings. Generalisability of the findings. Authors' comments on the strengths and weaknesses of the study. Likely action implication. Further research required.
Conclusion	Generalisability. Action implication.

Notwithstanding these difficulties, the appraisal must take place. After a thorough read of the research report, a written synopsis should be drawn up (Brown 1999). This needs to be based around a set of evaluative questions about the way the study was done. The process is in two inter-related parts. First, a set of descriptive information will need to be recorded. These include what its aims were, the type of study design, the sample and data collection methods. One is seemingly rewriting the report in a different format. Second, this information will need to be critically assessed to form a judgement about the quality of the way that the study was done. For example, interest will lie in whether or not there was adequate control of confounding variables, that is, other variables that could account for the study's results. Or, did the random allocation of individuals to the groups make them comparable at the beginning of the study? And if not, what else should have been done?

Key criteria for research studies

Whether interest lies in quantitative or qualitative research (see Chapter 2 for more information), the research study should meet three broad criteria. It should be:

- *Valid* – done well and generates good quality results.
- *Ethical* – undertaken according to acceptable and agreed moral/ethical standards and criteria.
- *Usable* – the findings and recommendations need to be relevant and feasible to implement in routine practice, ideally with the right level of detail.

The concept of research validity is central to the appraisal process. It provides the overarching research concept. At the same time, research studies must adhere to ethical standards, for example, at a minimum they must cover informed consent, anonymity and confidentiality (Long 1984). However, it is important to remember that ethical issues may arise at all stages in the study design, and thus its evaluation as well. This includes the reason why the research was undertaken on the topic (for example, was another study on this issue really needed?) to the take-up of valid research findings into practice. In addition, within the context of evidence-based practice, research findings should be relevant and implementable within routine practice (Long 1996). At its simplest, research should have an implication for action, at a practice and/or policy level.

In simple terms, something is valid if it measures what it is supposed to. Applied to a research study, the concept of research validity has two parts. First, there is the *internal validity* of the research. In essence, do the research results mean what they appear to? So, did the assumed causal variables lead to the observed results, or were the results *biased* and due to the effects of other uncontrolled extraneous factors? Second, there is *external validity*. Can the results be generalised, to other settings and to other populations? If a study has problematic internal validity, then there is no interest in generalisation.

A central part of the appraisal process will thus involve considering the possible threats to the internal validity of a study. Threats to internal validity may occur from three main sources:

1 Factors in the *selection* process, for example, due to the way the study subjects were chosen, the response rate and the settings selected ('selection' bias).

2 Factors in the measurement and observational process, for example, due to shortcomings in the definition and measurement of variables, data collection, coding and analysis ('information' bias).

3 The effects of uncontrolled, extraneous variables ('confounding') which could account for the study results.

A set of evaluative appraisal tools

Checklists to assist the appraisal of research reports are common place in any text on evidence-based practice (for example, Muir Gray 1997). Some, most notably those developed by the Critical Appraisal Skills Programme, are structured as a list of Yes–No type questions. These are available for randomised controlled trials, review studies and, most recently, qualitative studies. Others (for example, Brown 1999), while posed in question form, demand a textual commentary to elaborate on any identified difficulties. They make explicit the fact that the conclusions of any appraisal are judgemental. Strengths and weaknesses need to be identified. Notwithstanding these different forms, the value of either type lies in providing a systematic framework to follow through to assist in the critical appraisal.

The appraisal task may involve the review of a single study or of a set of studies. The material below takes the reader through some of the key appraisal questions outlined in Tables 3.1 and 3.2. Based around a set of methodological questions, the tool is intended to provide a comprehensive evaluation template. It purposely provides an extensive, yet informative and workable, series of questions to summarise the core content of the study and to assess the quality of the design in relation to its aims and outcomes. It aims to assist in thinking analytically, constructively and critically about the research study. For an example of a completed review using similar headings, see Appendix.

Table 3.1 A general evaluation tool/template

Review area	Review questions
Purpose	What are the aims of the study?
	What are the aims of the paper?
	Are these aims appropriate, given the state of knowledge in the area?
Study design	
Type of study	What type of study was used?
	Is the design appropriate given the aims and knowledge in the area?
Variables	What was studied?
	What were the intervention and any comparison intervention?
	Is sufficient detail provided to reproduce these?
Confounding	Are the effects of possible confounding variables controlled for?
	Do the authors take the effects of any uncontrolled confounders into consideration in the interpretation of the findings?
Measurement **	How are the variables measured? What are the outcome criteria?
	How valid and reliable is this measurement? Are the outcome measures responsive to change? Are the outcome measures appropriate and sufficiently broad to give insight into the perspectives of key stakeholders (patient, professional, service)? Can the measures be used in routine practice?

Table 3.1 Cont.

Review area	Review questions
	Was the follow-up time, if any, sufficient to warrant the conclusions drawn or to see the desired effects/outcomes?
Data collection	What data collection methods were used? Was there substantial measurement bias? What role did the researcher assume in doing the fieldwork? How were possible reactivity and subjectivity effects addressed? Was there substantial non-response? And loss to follow-up? Were the methods appropriate?
Sample and setting **	What is the setting and source population for the study participants? What are the inclusion and exclusion criteria? How and why were the study participants, and setting, chosen? Is the setting typical or representative of other settings and in what respects? If not, is this setting likely to present a stronger or weaker test of the research question? Is the sample of an adequate size to address the study's aims and to warrant its conclusions? Is the sample appropriate given the aims of the study?
Groups **	If the study has more than one group, how were study members allocated to each group? Were the groups of adequate size? Were the groups comparable? Were any important differences taken into account in the authors' analysis and interpretation of the findings?

Table 3.1 Cont.

Review area	Review questions
Conceptual and theoretical base	What is the underlying conceptual model or theoretical framework? What is the implied model of causal processes? In what way is this reflected in the measurements used? Do the authors address the possible contribution of their study to knowledge?
Ethics	Was Ethical Committee approval obtained? Was informed consent obtained from study participants? Are the findings presented so as to preserve the anonymity of informants? Have ethical issues been adequately addressed?
Study findings **	How was the data analysis undertaken? Do the findings fit with the authors' arguments and comments? Are the findings set in context with other findings in the area? How do they cohere with other research?
Policy and practice	To what setting are the study findings generalisable? To what population are the study's findings generalisable? Is the conclusion justified given the conduct of the study and any weaknesses identified? What contribution has the research made to knowledge? What are the implications for policy? What are the implications for service practice, and my own practice in particular?

Table 3.1 Cont.

Review area	Review questions
Summary evaluation	Looking across all the above areas, could the observed results have been brought about by something other than the intervention/variables studied?
	In summary, what are the strengths and weaknesses of the study?
	What further research may be required? What major gaps in knowledge remain?
	What are possible theory, policy and practice implications?
	What have I learned?

** Areas where questions to appraise qualitative studies substantially diverge (see Table 3.2).

A single evaluation tool cannot do justice to the multiplicity of different research designs. These will embrace quantitative designs, ranging from a survey to a randomised controlled trial, qualitative designs and systematic reviews. As each type of study has different features, the exact questions asked must vary. For example, in reviewing a randomised controlled trial it is important to identify and comment on the form of random allocation used (see the Consort Statement, Altman 1996).

This is most problematic, however, in the context of the appraisal of qualitative researchers. Indeed, the feasibility, and even appropriateness, of the task is hotly contested (Denzin 1994; but see Murphy *et al.* 1998 for a comprehensive review and approach). At the same time, within the context of evidence-based practice, if qualitative research is going to play its rightful role, the quality of qualitative studies must be assessed. A transparency over the way the study is done is needed. Otherwise, for example, it is difficult to convince others that the findings are not simply anecdotal, instead of being based on a rigorous and systematic approach, linking data, description and interpretation.

Even more problematic is the fact that within the qualitative tradition there is no single definition of, or approach to, qualitative research. But one must be cognisant of the fact that quantitative and qualitative research is based on different epistemologies. They also employ different methodological concepts in describing the research style. In this light, to supplement the general evaluation tool, Table 3.2 presents some modified questions for qualitative research, picking up the specific areas asterisked in Table 3.1.

Table 3.2 Areas where questions to appraise qualitative studies substantially diverge: modifications of the evaluation tool for qualitative research

Review area	Review questions
Setting	Within what geographical and care setting is the study carried out?
	What is the rationale for and appropriateness of choosing this setting?
	Is sufficient detail given about the setting?
	Over what time period is the study conducted?
	Is this sufficient?
Sample	How is the sample (informants, settings and events) selected?
	What is the size of the study sample and groups forming the study?
	Is the sample appropriate in terms of depth (intensity of data collection – individuals, settings and events) and width across time, settings and events (does it capture key persons and events)?
	Is the sample (informants, settings and events) appropriate to the aims of the study?
Data collection	What data collection methods are used to obtain and record the data? Are these appropriate?
	Are the data available for inspection/independent analysis?

Table 3.2 Cont.

Review area	Review questions
	What role does the researcher adopt within the setting?
	Is the process of fieldwork adequately described, for example, in terms of an account of how the data were elicited; the type and range of questions; an interview guide; the length and timing of observation work; and process of field-note taking?
Data analysis	How are the data analysed?
	How adequate is the description of the data analysis? Is sufficient detail given to allow for its reproduction? Are adequate steps taken to guard against selectivity in selecting data for presentation in the study report?
	Is adequate evidence provided to support the analysis? For example, does it include original/raw data extracts? Are there indications of iterative analysis? Is the presented evidence representative? What efforts are made to establish its validity, such as searching for negative evidence, use of multiple sources and checking back with informants?
	Is the study set in a broader context, in terms of findings and relevant theory?
Researcher bias	Are the researcher's own position, assumptions and possible biases outlined?
	How could these have affected the study, in particular, the analysis and interpretation of the data?

Appraising research is not an 'exact' science, or rather methodology. It remains for the appraiser to come to a judgement about whether the study, or part of its findings, is sufficiently credible to be taken into the knowledge base and taken into practice. Any apparent Yes–No type question needs to be amplified with an account of why and the issues raised.

What were the study's aims?

The beginning point of any critical appraisal, whatever the study design, must be the identification of the aims of the study. At one level, this may seem a straightforward, descriptive question, but unfortunately it often is not. The authors may indicate the aims of their broader research rather than the particular parts that they are reporting on in this article. Or, the article may seem to address issues other than those that the authors indicate. The fact that the aims are not made clear early on in the paper (one would expect this in the introduction section) just makes things a little more difficult for the appraiser. It does not make the study any less valuable. Whatever, the appraiser will need to reflect on what the authors indicate. Does their stated aim adequately cover the material reported in the study? If not, how can the aims be better phrased?

What type of study was used?

Closely following identification of the study's aims, it is sensible to identify the type of study design that was used. Is it a cross-sectional survey, a randomised controlled trial or a qualitative study based on participant observation? While nomenclature in the research field is often cumbersome, the appraiser should use phrases that describe the study best and in ways that their colleagues are familiar with.

The value of identifying the type of design is to alert the appraiser to the expected strengths and weaknesses of the design. These can provide useful pointers of what to look for. For example, in a randomised controlled trial, one of the first things to check is whether the randomisation has worked: that is, are the two (or more) groups similar at the start of the study? Or, within a survey design, was the sample representative? A later question is whether an alternative study design might have been more appropriate to use, either to cast light on the particular research aims or given the current state of knowledge in the area.

What was studied?

This leads straightforwardly into summarising what was studied. What variables were explored, what was the intervention and any comparative intervention? From an evaluation perspective, interest lies in the level of detail provided. Was it sufficient to enable reproduction of the intervention within your own practice? An associated question, at least for quantitative studies, relates to the way that the variables were measured. Issues of reliability and validity are central. Again, it is a question of describing what the authors did and reflecting on its quality.

Within a qualitative study, at a descriptive level, interest lies in identifying the data collection methods used to obtain and record the data and clarifying the role that the researcher adopted in the setting. Issues of reactivity (how the informants may have responded to the presence and queries of the researcher) and subjectivity (how the researcher chose what, who, when and how to collect data) provide core foci for the evaluation. Indeed, it is critical to try to identify the researcher's own views of the topic area, assumptions made and possible biases, thinking on how these could affect the data collection, analysis and interpretation of the data. Thus, were the processes of data collection and recording adequately described and appropriate?

These issues are intertwined in a qualitative study with the way the data are analysed due to the expected constant interplay between data collection and analysis. Again, moving beyond the simple description of how the data were analysed (for example, searching for categories and themes based on the informants' perceptions), the appraiser must come to a conclusion over whether adequate evidence is provided to support the analysis. For example, are original quotations provided? Are these and descriptions of events representative (or highly selective)? Has the researcher demonstrated efforts to establish the validity of their analysis by searching for negative examples or using multiple data sources?

Where was the study undertaken and with whom?

A further set of questions relates to where the study was undertaken, that is, the study setting and sample. For a quantitative study, interest lies in the appropriateness of the inclusion and exclusion criteria, the sample selection method, sample size and implications of any loss to follow-up. The same questions have relevance to a systematic review. Here though, the interpretation of 'sample' relates to the number of databases searched, and sample size to the number of studies included in the review. If the study involves more than one group of subjects, further issues will relate to the way study members were allocated to groups.

Within a qualitative study, there is greater interest in the setting, the detail provided upon it and its appropriateness as a context to explore the study aims. This arises because of the focus of qualitative research in trying to illuminate the meanings attached by individuals to events and situations, from different perspectives and bounded by the context or setting within which events are located. Further, the notion of 'sample' needs to be interpreted in a broader manner; not just informants, but also settings and events. Evaluative questions will explore the appropriateness of the sample in terms of its depth (the intensity of data collection) and width across time, settings and events.

What is the underlying conceptual and theoretical framework?

Sometimes studies do not make plain an underlying theoretical or conceptual framework. The study seemingly has only an empirical bent. Others are very specific, contextualising the study within the broader theoretical literature. For the appraiser, knowing where the researcher is coming from can be very informative in appraising a piece of research. Their approach may unfortunately have blinded them to the possibility of an alternative explanation of the data, or the need to control for a particular variable, or to explore the implications/relevance of a particular situation on their emerging theory.

How are potential ethical issues addressed?

Too often ethical issues in research are left implicit. Any evaluation of a research study should pay close attention to the way that the research has ensured that the study members, at a minimum, have come to no harm by participating in the study and, more appropriately, that they will benefit from such participation. The practice of research and associated ethical issues are more commonly discussed in terms of the balance of societal benefit and individual harm (Sapsford and Evans 1979).

For the research appraiser, it is important to remember that ethical research is more than just questions over informed consent, confidentiality and anonymity. For example, was the study needed? That is, was there sufficient evidence in this area such that management and practice action should already have taken the findings on board?

How do the findings cohere with other studies?

Any research study should be expected to add to knowledge. This may relate to knowledge about a particular setting, the appropriateness of a particular research method in addressing the topic area, or wider theory and/or understanding. The appraiser will be examining the extent to which the report's author(s) have set their findings in the context of other research in the area. At a minimum, it is necessary to comment on the extent to which the findings link back to the aims of the study.

What are the policy and practice implications?

Once there is sufficient confidence about the internal validity of the study, that is, its strengths outweigh its weaknesses, interest must turn to potential action implications of the findings. These will most commonly be closely surrounded by caveats, to take account of the inevitable weaknesses of the study, themselves arising as a *sine qua non* of research in practice. In the context of evidence-based practice, with interest lying in the potential implementation of the findings in *my* practice, emphasis lies on thinking through whether the findings are generalisable to other settings and populations.

Most directly, the interest is in 'how could my practice be changed?' based on these findings. Brown (1999: 112) most usefully raises two further questions:

How should I go about making the change?

Once I change my practice, how will I know if patients have benefited?

While these issues are outside of the narrow vein of appraising research, they bring attention full-circle back to its core purpose within the context of evidence-based practice, namely, using appropriate research findings in practice. The practitioner will need to set up a process of measurement to monitor whether or not the desired outcomes are being achieved (Long 1997).

Summarising the appraisal and putting it all together

Once the evaluation of the article is complete, there is considerable value in drawing together a summary of the appraisal. This should be your response to the question, 'Is there anything about the way the study was done that may . . . deter you from applying the findings into practice?' Thus, in summary, what are the strengths and weaknesses of the study? And, what are possible theory, policy and practice implications? A further useful question is: 'what have I learned from this study?' (Sapsford and Evans 1979). This could relate to the topic area or methodology/the practice of research.

Particular modifications for qualitative research

In leading the reader through the general evaluation tool, attention was drawn to a number of modifications to the questions and areas to take account of the philosophy and practice of qualitative research. Table 3.2 does this more explicitly. Primary focus lies on the plausibility and credibility of the findings in the context of the way the study was undertaken. Issues of potential reactivity, to the researcher, and subjectivity, by the researcher, are central (in a quantitative vernacular, these are examples of potential measurement biases). So, too, are factors relating to the choice of setting and informants (sampling) and ways to enhance confidence in the findings through triangulation of data sources, multiple perspectives and points of observation, theoretical sampling and use of the constant comparative method. Critical points of contrast lie in sections on setting and sample and data analysis. Particular attention lies in 'why this setting?', 'why these informants or events?' and 'are key events and informants captured?'. Interest lies in explicating the context of the informants' experiences and accounts. Contrasts lie in the depth and width of the sample and an interpretation of the sample in terms of persons, places and events. This compares to the quantitative research style's emphasis on sample size and representation. In the analysis context, the potential threat of researcher subjectivity needs to be addressed: that is, what is seen, heard, recorded, and then recognised in the analysis and interpretation of the data. For example, interest lies, *inter alia*, on evidence of iterative analysis and the presentation of representative evidence showing supporting and contrary data to any theoretical account arising.

Conclusion

'Doing critical appraisal' requires use of a systematic approach. The evaluation tool outlined in this chapter provides a framework of questions to enable this. The tool aims to provide a structure to both describe and evaluate the characteristics of the study (for example, study type, sampling and setting) and how the study was done (rationale for the choice of setting, sample, data collection and analysis). It should act as an aide and learning tool. Moreover, it may provide a means to communicate your evaluation to others. Indeed, the evaluation tool could be utilised in the form of a database. This would assist in developing a pool of evaluated studies, around a common framework of review areas.

In the author's own research reviews, this is the approach adopted (HCPRDU 1998). The database record provided the research team's source document, avoiding the necessity of returning to the article.

It is thus essential that the descriptive and evaluative comments for each question or database field are self-standing. Use of a more simplistic dichotomous (Yes–No) response must be avoided, even if the question can be so answered. The aim is to facilitate explanation. The evaluative comments are, in principle and in practice, informed judgements, based on the detail provided in the study report.

In a database format, the evaluation tool needs a user friendly front end. The approach has been to separate a number of key aspects from the main body of the evaluation, namely:

● Purpose/aims of the study and aims of the paper.
● Key findings.
● Summary evaluative comments.

The result forms a simplified, evaluative abstract. Its purpose is to enable the appraiser and any subsequent reader of the review quickly to grasp the essential details of a study and its potential value. Within the context of evidence-based practice, to this could valuably be added:

● Summary implications for changing practice.

The checklist outlined in this chapter has been tried, tested and modified within teaching and research. It is purposely elaborative and discouraging of Yes–No responses. Whether it should be simplified to encourage wide use by busy practitioners is crucial. The critical appraisal of research is not just a question of judging that the study is of 'poor' or 'good' quality and relevance to policy and/or practice. Constructive evaluation requires an explanation of how and why this judgement was arrived at and, in other contexts, ways to overcome any identified weaknesses.

Evaluating studies, be they qualitative or quantitative, involves a process of judgement. An intended consequence of the use of a systematic checklist is to reduce the variation in judgements and opinions about the quality and relevance of a study. To this end, adequate knowledge, skill and training is required of the relevant methodologies and problems and the difficulties faced in their execution. Educational and training events, such as the Critical Appraisal Skills Programme in the UK or the Canadian

McMasters approach to teaching evidence-based practice, have an important role to play in this regard.

Finally, it is perhaps reasonable to ask the question 'why is critical appraisal so important?' especially for peer reviewed journals. Certainly, peer review makes a difference. But problematic articles are still published in good quality peer reviewed journals. More widely, not all journals are peer reviewed. In the longer term and thinking optimistically, the answer ought to be that the findings of poorly designed and executed studies will not published. For the good studies that are published, all that may remain is to judge the potential relevance of the study's findings for one's own setting and the feasibility of implementing them. But this is only a possible future!

Summary of key points

● Critical appraisal is the foundation for evidence-informed practice.
● Successful critical appraisal requires the adoption of systematic framework.
● Critical appraisal requires an understanding and appreciation of the reliability and validity issues associated with either quantitative or qualitative research.

Recommended reading

Crombie, I.K. (1996) *The Pocket Guide to Critical Appraisal* London, BMJ Publishing Group.
Useful Web Site: <http://www.nzgg.org.nz

References

Altman, D.G. (1996) Better reporting of randomised controlled trials: the CONSORT statement, *British Medical Journal* 313, 570–1.

Brown S.J. (1999) *Knowledge for Healthcare Practice* Philadelphia, WB Saunders Co.

Denzin, N.K. (1994) The art and politics of interpretation. In Denzin, N.K. and Lincoln, Y.S. (eds) *Handbook of Qualitative Research*, London, Sage, 500–15.

Froom, P. and Froom, J. (1993) Deficiencies in structured medical abstracts, *Journal of Clinical Epidemiology* 46, 7, 591–4.

Haynes, R.B. (1993) More informative abstracts: Current status and evaluation, *Journal of Clinical Epidemiology* 46, 7, 595–7.

HCPRDU (1998) <http://www.fhsc.salford.ac.uk/heprdu/assessment.htm>

Long, A.F. (1984) *Research into Health and Illness*, Aldershot, Gower Publishing Co Ltd.

Long, A.F. (1996) Health services research – A radical approach to cross the research and development divide? In Baker, M. and Kirk, S. (eds) *Research and Development for the NHS* 51–64, Abingdon, Radcliffe Medical Press Ltd.

Long, A.F. and Harrison, S. (1996) Evidence-based decision-making, *Health Services Journal*, Glaxo Wellcome Supplement, Issue 6 (11 January), 1–12.

Long, A.F. (1997) Key issues in outcomes measurement, *International Journal of STD and AIDS* 8, 663–7.

McSherry, R. (1997) What do registered nurses and midwives feel and know about research? *Journal of Advanced Nursing* 25, 985–98.

Muir Gray, J.A. (1997) *Evidence-Based Health Care* Edinburgh, Churchill Livingstone.

Murphy, E., Dingwall, R., Greatbatch D., Parker, S. and Watson, P. (1998) Qualitative research methods in health technology assessment: A review of the literature, *Health Technology Assessment* 2, 16.

Narine, L., Yee, D.S., Eimarson, T.R. and Ilersiclo, A.L. (1991) Quality of abstracts of original research articles in CMAJ in 1989, *Canadian Medical Association Journal* 144, 449–53.

Rosenberg, W. and Donald, A. (1995) Evidence-based medicine: An approach to clinical problem solving, *British Medical Journal* 310, 1122–6.

Sackett, D.L., Rosenberg, W., Muir Gray, J.A., Haynes, R.B. and Richardson, W.S. (1996a) Evidence-based medicine: What it is and what it isn't, *British Medical Journal* 312, 71–2.

Sackett, D.L., Richardson, W.S., Rosenberg, W. and Haynes, R.B. (1996b) *How to Practise and Teach Evidence-Based Medicine* Edinburgh, Churchill Livingstone.

Sapsford, R.J. and Evans, J. (1979) *Evaluation of Research*, DE304, Research Methods in Education and the Social Sciences, Block 8, Milton Keynes, Open University Press.

Stern, P.C. (1979) *Evaluating Social Science Research* New York, Oxford University Press.

Chapter 4
Benefits of research to nursing practice

Maxine Simmons

Introduction

This chapter is concerned with the benefits of using research findings in nursing care. The benefits of utilising research in improving patient care will be explored. Some may argue that research is an academic process of interest to nurses in education or research and essential if undertaking a course, but which has no real place in the reality of nursing care delivery. However, the *raison d'être* of research in nursing is 'to improve the quality of patient care and to increase the effectiveness and efficiency of the nursing service (Tierney 1991). The purpose of this chapter is to demonstrate how research findings can be of benefit in nursing practice.

Evidence-informed care in context

For research to be of benefit it needs 'to do good', to 'improve upon' current practice. Research has a significant role to play in improving nursing care as much of nursing practice remains rooted in myth and traditional ritual, with nurses acting in the ways they do because 'this is the way it has always been done' (Ford and Walsh 1989). For research to be of benefit the nurse needs to perceive the research as being of use in improving their practice. This is perhaps a logical starting point as not all research is valid, reliable or suitable for all areas of clinical practice. Chapter 3 discussed the necessity to review the research findings critically, but, to date, how much benefit have research findings been to practice? Despite the fact that research has been on the nursing profession's agenda for some time, only a moderate proportion of nurses use research as a basis for practice. To resolve this we need to understand where nursing research fits with nursing knowledge and subsequent practices.

The following case study demonstrates an area of practice where particular research findings were evaluated and thought not to be of benefit to a specific client group. It demonstrates the use of different types of knowledge by the nurses.

Case study 4.1

A nurse who had recently been employed in a spinal injuries unit was concerned about the management of catheter care on the ward. It was routine that at night patients would disconnect their catheter from their 'leg bag' and attach an overnight drainage bag. This practice was thereby, breaking the closed seal-drainage system.

In the light of research findings, let us explore the potential benefits to nursing practice.

There is substantial evidence from a number of research studies demonstrating that disconnection of the closed-seal urinary drainage system increases the risk of the development of urinary tract infections (Gillespie *et al.* 1964, Garibaldi *et al.* 1974, Platt *et al.* 1982).

Following discussions with the ward team, the nurse was informed that the staff were aware of the research relating to catheters and urinary tract infections; however, they felt it was inappropriate to implement (maintaining a closed-seal drainage system) this practice for patients with spinal injuries. Patients on the unit were aware of the need to maintain an empty bladder. (Maintaining an empty bladder for patients who have spinal injuries and neuropathic bladders (the bladder lacks 'sensation') is necessary because if the bladder is allowed to become full, they risk developing neurogenic shock and being in a life threatening situation very quickly.)

The patients on the spinal injuries unit took great care to avoid developing neurogenic shock by ensuring that their catheter would drain unrestricted overnight. They did not trust the system of attaching the 'leg bag' to the overnight drainage bag, as their experience was that this can result in 'kinking' of the tubing, preventing drainage from the 'leg bag' with the consequence of a full bladder. The patients had made an informed choice to increase their risk of developing urinary tract infections rather than risk the development of neurogenic shock.

To understand the actions of the nurses in the case study it would seem relevant to explore the knowledge base(s) the nurses used to underpin their clinical decisions. This can be explained as described by Carper (1978), who identified four fundamental ways of knowing in nursing. These are as follows:

- Empirics – the science of nursing.
- Aesthetics – the art of nursing.
- Personal knowledge.
- Ethics.

In relation to the case study, the reality of the situation is that the patient care situation was complex and the care decisions could not be based on technical-rational knowledge alone (Schon 1987). Research knowledge should not be implemented to the exclusion of other types of knowledge, else nursing care would be at risk of being mechanical and non-therapeutic. To practise evidence-informed nursing in this situation 'nurses require clinical expertise, resources and research evidence together with an understanding of the patient preference' (Cullum *et al.* 1998). Therefore research needs to be considered in the light of individual circumstances if it is to be of benefit. The variables of each unique situation, and the outcome of the evidence-informed action in relation to the benefit for the individual as a whole, need to be considered to promote the delivery of holistic care (Keegan 1987).

Benner (1984) discusses the concept of knowledge embedded in expertise. Nurses must develop the knowledge base (know-how) for practice, through scientific investigation and observation, to begin to develop the know-how of clinical expertise. In this sense, theory is developed from practice, and then practice can be altered or extended by theory rather than vice versa.

Case study 4.2 provides an example of expert nurses adjusting a research-based practice to meet the unique needs of individual patients.

Case study 4.2

A nurse working on a urology ward had read an article, which described an experimental research study involving patients, post-transurethral (via the urethra) surgery.

The research involved comparing the micturition patterns and length of time to discharge of patients who had their catheters removed at 6am (control group) or 12 midnight (experimental group). The traditional practice on the ward was to remove catheters at 6am for trial without catheter following transurethral surgery.

In the light of the research findings let us explore the potential benefits to nursing practice.

The research findings by Noble *et al.* (1990), Crowe *et al.* (1994) and Chillington (1992) demonstrated that patients who had their catheters removed at 12 midnight voided larger amounts of urine at first void, the time to first void was greater and patients were discharged home earlier than the control group.

Following a review of the above research literature and a trial period to evaluate the practice of removing catheters at 12 midnight, the ward changed to the practice of midnight catheter removal for all patients requiring trial without catheter. After a period of time it became evident that experienced nurses were adjusting the time of catheter removal based on the individual patient's needs, that is, when the patient was ready to go to bed rather than 12 midnight. Occasionally, the nurse who had been on night duty reported that a patient had been anxious about having their catheter removed before going to sleep and that some patients feared that they might not wake if they needed to pass urine. Nurses' responses to these situations varied, with more experienced nurses allowing the patient informed choice and, where the patient remained anxious, leaving the catheter in place until the morning.

The case studies demonstrate that for research findings to be of benefit to patients the nurse requires not only knowledge of the available research, but also an understanding of the individual patient's psychological status and social circumstances as well as their physical condition. This approach of considering individual patient circumstances in the application of research findings is supported by Sackett *et al.* (1996). Sackett's definition of evidence-based medicine emphasises the need to blend evidence with clinical expertise in order to decide if, and how, the evidence might relate to the individual patient.

On reflection, when considering implementing the above research findings, it would have been beneficial to think about the implications the change might have had on some patients' psychological status and social situation. For example :

- The issue of incontinence during the night is probably a significant fear for many patients following prostate surgery, considering that they will most likely have suffered nocturia for several years.
- The issue of early discharge may be important for many patients, although some patients may have delayed discharge, despite a successful trial without catheter, due to requiring social support.

The 12 midnight catheter removal research undoubtedly reduces length of hospital stay for many patients; however, the research itself has limitations of its validity and reliability as the sample sizes in all the studies were small. The samples used were limited to only one ward in both studies, therefore the findings cannot be generalised to all urology patients as other variables, that is, surgical technique, cannot be excluded.

> **Box 4.1 For research findings to be of benefit a nurse needs to:**
>
> - view the research findings critically;
> - consider the appropriateness of the research for their unique clinical area and individual patients;
> - utilise other sources of knowledge whilst implementing evidence-based nursing;
> - recognise that not all effective decisions are research based.

From the above it would appear that the primary goal of nursing research is to develop a scientific knowledge base for nursing practice. Hegyvary (1991) states that a solid research base will provide evidence of the nursing actions that are effective in promoting positive patient outcomes. Case study 4.3 provides an example of a common patient problem and suggests an evidence-informed intervention which is of more benefit than the commonly implemented medical treatment.

To improve the management of constipation, nurses need to look beyond the medical model of prescription medicines and plan nurse-led interventions to enable the patient to regain control of their bowel function as part of their rehabilitation towards independence.

A systematic review ('A literature review that has been prepared using a systematic approach. It seeks to identify and synthesises all the literature on an given topic', Nelson 1998: 24) of the treatment of constipation revealed that laxatives do work and on average

Case study 4.3

Constipation is a frequently recorded problem on patient care plans in hospital. This is perhaps not surprising as constipation may affect up to 20 per cent of people aged over 65 years (Rouse *et al.* 1991) and the results of one study of constipation demonstrated an incidence for older people of 79 per cent in hospitals, 59 per cent in nursing homes and 38 per cent in people living at home (Kinnunen 1991). The common nursing intervention to prevent constipation is to administer medically prescribed aperients, although the consequence of using aperients has been suggested to do more harm than failing to have the bowels open daily (Heading 1987).

(mean) increase bowel movements from 3.5 to 5 per week. However, for adult patients with constipation bran or bulk laxatives work as well as anything, and advising patients with chronic constipation to eat more fruit and vegetables and have some bran seems to be the best advice on the evidence available (Tramonte *et al.* 1997).

The following care plan has been adapted from a long-term management of constipation protocol compiled following a comprehensive literature search by Wood *et al.* (1995). The care plan below suggests evidence-informed nursing interventions as the first-line management of constipation of a fictitious patient.

In summary, the benefits of using research findings in practice is that it can facilitate improved patient outcomes by informing nurses of alternative interventions which have been proven to be more beneficial.

The outlined case studies highlight the benefits of using research to enable both individual and teams of nurses to use it to improve care for each individual patient. It is also important to demonstrate how the standardisation of research findings can be of benefit not only to individual patients, but also to patients' groups and health care organisations by the application of integrated care pathways.

Patient problem	Goal	Intervention	Evaluation
John is at risk of developing constipation following his CVA.	John will pass a soft stool at least every two days. (Rationale – 7% of men defecate 3 times daily and 40% of men defecate once daily (Heaton et al. 1992).	1 Maintain fluid intake at more than 2 litres a day (assist John with eating and drinking). 2 Increase mobility (assist John with mobilising to the toilet rather than using the commode or urinals). 3 Increase fibre in diet (advise John to eat at least three portions of fruit or vegetables per day and select high fibre options from meal menus, i.e. bran-based cereals and brown bread). 4 Ensure private toileting to promote patient privacy.	

Integrated care pathways

Integrated care pathways (also known as co-ordinated care pathways, care maps or anticipated care pathways) are task orientated care plans which detail essential steps in the care of patients with a specific clinical problem and describe the patient's expected clinical course (Coffey *et al.* 1992, Kitchner and Bundred 1996). They offer a structured means of developing and implementing local protocols of care based on evidence. They provide a means of identifying the reason why clinical care falls short of the adopted standard through supplying data identifying patients who did not receive the care described in the pathway or whose outcome was not that antici-pated (Campbell *et al.* 1998).

The process of developing an integrated care pathway requires that the professionals involved (and this should involve all disci-plines who deliver care to patients with the chosen condition for the pathway) select clinical conditions where variations in practice occur and affect patient outcome. Through using research to develop integrated care pathways, practice becomes standardised to that which is demonstrated to be the most clinically and cost effec-tive (Campbell *et al.* 1998). Grimshaw *et al.* (1995) have demonstrated that the use of evidence-based clinical guidelines has improved patient care.

Campbell *et al.* (1998) state that although integrated care path-ways can be a strategy for implementing evidence-informed care to improve patient outcomes, they do have some disadvantages. They are time consuming to create, may discourage the use of profes-sional judgement in individual circumstances or innovation and are difficult to develop in diseases which have less predictable path-ways and outcomes, that is, mental health.

Holland (1998) describes how the implementation of an Integrated Care Pathway (ICP) for patients admitted for Transurethral Resection of Prostate (TURP) facilitates:

- Patient involvement – through the ICP being visible on the end of the patient's bed and the ICP being discussed with the patient on admission so they can see what to expect, and patients are encouraged to take part in their care as an individual rather than as part of the process.
- Enhances uni-professional and multi-professional communi-cation – through providing a clear written plan of what has to be achieved each day and any variation from the ICP, plus the reason for that variance, is documented. Encourages dis-cussion between medical and nursing staff regarding variances.
- Enables multi-professional decision-making as nurses are able to make decisions on variances rather than waiting for a doctor.
- Ensures consistency of care and assists in risk reduction through maintaining a tight control on treatment interventions

and if new doctors want to do something different, they have to record it.

- Allows comparison of the efficiency of clinicians by comparing patients' median length of stay.
- Aids cost efficiency as treatment regimens can be amended as a result of analysis of the variance data.
- Provides data which can be used as a basis for audit and research.

Summary

The benefits of using research in care plans and integrated care pathways to both groups of patients and organisations are as follows:

- potential reduction in litigation through implementing safest practice and evidence-based protocols;
- achievement of the aims and objectives of clinical governance through practitioners who are able to demonstrate they are practising as accountable clinicians who base their decisions on evidence rather than ritual, and achieve the standards for practice as determined by NICE and CHI (McSherry and Haddock 1999);
- best use of resources through implementing practices which are demonstrated to be the most clinical and cost effective interventions.

Conclusion

In the light of the discussions surrounding the value of research to individual patients and healthcare organisations, the future is undoubtedly an exciting time for nursing. Ritual and traditional practices need to be replaced by individualised care based on sound knowledge. Patients will benefit from the ability of nurses to integrate best evidence with professional judgements to produce packages of care which result in effective personalised nursing interventions. The development of standardised evidenced-based protocols/guidelines will ensure the implementation of practices based on best evidence. The continual auditing of these practices will promote clinical effectiveness, reduce clinical risk and meet the objectives of Clinical Governance.

Summary of key points

- Evidence-informed nursing is achievable in everyday clinical practice.
- Integrated care pathways, protocols and core care plans can enable a structured approach to the use of research and the standardisation of nursing care.

Recommended reading

Benner, P. (1984) *From Novice to Expert Excellence and Power in Clinical Nursing Practice* Califormia, Addison

Carper, B.A. (1978) Fundamental patterns of knowing in nursing, *Advances In Nursing Science* 1, 1, 13–23

References

Benner, P. (1984) *From Novice to Expert Excellence and Power in Clinical Nursing Practice* California, Addison Wesley.

Campbell, H., Hotchkiss, R., Bradshaw, N. and Porteous, M. (1998) Integrated care pathways, *British Medical Journal* 316, Jan, 133–7.

Carper, B.A. (1978) Fundamental patterns of knowing in nursing, *Advances In Nursing Science* 1, 1, 13–23.

Chillington, B. (1992) Early removal advances discharge home, *Professional Nurse* Nov, 82–9.

Coffey, R., Richards, J., Remment, C., Leroy, S., Schoville, R. and Baldwin, P. An introduction to critical paths, *Quality Management in Health Care* 75, 45–54.

Crowe, H., Clift, R. and Bolton, D. (1994) Randomised study of the effect of midnight removal of urinary catheters, *Urology Nursing* 14, 18–20.

Cullum, N., Dicenso, A. and Ciliska, D. (1998) Implementing evidence-based nursing: Some misconceptions, *Evidence-Based Medicine* 1, 2, 38–40.

Ford, M. and Walsh, P. (1989) *Nursing Rituals: Research and Rational Actions* Oxford, Butterworth Heinemann.

Garibaldi, R.A. *et al.* (1974) Factors predisposing to bacteriuria during indwelling catheterisation, *The New England Journal of Medicine* 291, 5, 215–19.

Gillespie, W.A. *et al.* (1964) Prevention of urinary infection in gynaecology patients, *British Medical Journal* 2, 423–5.

Grimshaw, J., Freemantle, N., Wallace, S., Russell, I., Hurwitz, B., Watt, I., Long, A. and Sheldon, T. (1995) Developing and implementing clinical practice guidelines, *Quality In Health Care* 4, 190–93.

Heading, C. (1987) Nursing assessment and management of constipation *Nursing: The Journal of Clinical Practice, Education and Management* 3, 21, Sept, 778–80.

Heaton, K.W., Radvan, H. and Cripps, H. (1992) Defecation frequency and timing and stool form in the general population: A prospective study, *Gut* 33, 818–24.

Hegyvary, S.T. (1991) Issues in outcomes research, *Journal of Nursing Quality Assurance* 5, 2, 1–6.

Holland, M. (1998) Keep to the path and save cash, *Medical Interface* April, 27–8.

Keegan, L. (1987) Holistic nursing, *American Operating Room Nurses Journal* 46, 499–506.

Kinnunen, O. (1991) Study of constipation in a geriatric hospital, day hospital, old people's home and at home, *Ageing* 3, 2, 161–70.

Kitchner, D. and Bundred, P. (1996) Integrated care pathways, *Archives of Disease in Childhood* 75, 166–8.

McSherry, R. and Haddock, J. (1999) Linking the key components, *Clinical Governance Health Care Risk Report* April, 14–16.

Nelson, E.A. (1998) The value of systematic reviews in research, *Professional Nurse* 14, 1, October, 24–8.

Noble, J.G., Menzies, D., Cox, P.J. and Edwards, L. (1990) Midnight removal: An improved approach to removal of catheters, *British Journal of Urology* 65, 615–17.

Platt, R. *et al.* (1982) Mortality associated with nosocomial urinary tract infection, *New England Journal of Medicine* 307, 11, 637–41.

Rouse, M., Mahapatra, M., Atkinson, S.M. and Prescott, P. (1991) An open randomised parallel group study of lactulose versus ispaghula in the treatment of chronic constipation in adults, *British Journal of Clinical Practice* 45, 28–30.

Sackett, L.D., Rosenburg, W. and Haynes, B.R. (1996) *Evidence Based Medicine: How to Practise and Teach EBM* London, Churchill Livingstone.

Schon, D. (ed.) (1987) *Educating the Reflective Practitioner* San Francisco, Jossey Bass.

Tierney, A.J. (1991) Ch. 32, p. 331. In Cormack D.F.S. (ed.) *The Research Process in Nursing*, 2nd edn, Part 3, Oxford, Blackwell Scientific Publications.

Tramonte, S.M., Brand, N.B. and Mulrow, C.D. *et al.* (1997) The treatment of chronic constipation: A systematic review, *Journal of General Internal Medicine* 12, 15–24.

Wood, S.I., Kay, C.A., Hayton, B., Kaye, A., Bunn, D. and Corracle, O.J. (1995) Are health professionals guilty of laxative abuse? *The Pharmaceutical Journal* 255, 11, Nov, 659–61.

Chapter 5

Reflective practice and decision-making related to research implementation

Jane Haddock

CONTENTS

Introduction

This chapter will consider reflective practice and decision-making and discuss how the nurse may use this professional knowledge in conjunction with evidence-based literature in the delivery of everyday clinical care. The aim of the chapter is to provide the reader with guidance to enable them to correctly identify the problem with which they are faced in order to select the right evidence-based intervention for the situation.

Nursing requires complex decision-making (Benner 1984) in relation to providing care where nurses are required to make clinical and managerial decisions as part of their everyday work. They are faced with the complexity of individual patients and working within a team of staff in a multi-professional organisation.

The importance of developing and using research evidence to inform all aspects of decision-making in health care has been emphasised in the previous chapters.

This chapter builds upon this by exploring:

- elements of clinical expertise;
- problem solving;
- the assessment process;
- clinical decision-making models;
- reflective practice.

This chapter aims to develop readers' knowledge and understanding of these elements to enable them to integrate decision-making processes and reflective practice skills in the application of evidence into practice.

Clinical expertise

We can all name those nurses who are regarded as 'experts' in their particular clinical area. These particular nurses keep up to date with knowledge and relevant skills, and both deliver and evaluate the care they give.

Expertise develops when nurses test and refine propositions, hypotheses and principles based on expectations in actual practice (Benner 1984). Within nursing, the expert has been described as having the ability to gain a perceptual grasp of a problem *only* in the light of a patient's past history and within the context of the current situation (Polanyi 1958, cited in Benner 1984). Polanyi describes this ability as 'connoisseurship' and a key feature in the recognitional ability of the expert.

The main features in clinical expertise are:

- reflecting on clinical practice;
- having the ability to learn from previous experiences;
- having the skill to assess patients within their current context;
- collecting the appropriate information;
- understanding the meaning of the information collected;
- formulating a problem and judging its significance and relationship with others;
- making a clinical decision within the context of the individual patient's situation;
- evaluating practice to establish effectiveness.

(Carpenito 1989, Hurst *et al.* 1991, Haynes *et al.* 1996)

Clinical expertise is therefore an important feature in the process of evidence-informed decision-making. Although some decisions are straightforward and require little or no expertise to guarantee a favourable outcome, others require skilled judgement to identify the problem and intervene effectively.

In order to intervene effectively, identifying the problem is the most critical stage in the decision-making process. If the problem or diagnosis formulated is erroneous, then the subsequent decision and plan of intervention will also be in error. For example, if a nurse does not have the ability to establish whether a terminally ill patient is experiencing pain or not, neither analgesia for the pain nor complementary interventions will occur, and thus this lack will have an effect on the pain management of the patient. Thus, the evidence on the management of terminal pain from systematic reviews or meta analysis will be of little use for that patient.

Problem solving

Evidence-informed decision-making involves the identification of the problem(s) and deciding the best way to solve it, informed by evidence of effectiveness, patient's preference and the resources available in practice. To foster a systematic approach to decision-making, nurses have adopted a problem-solving model to organise their work. Within nursing the approach has been informed by the 'Stages Model Theory' of problem solving (Hurst *et al.* 1991).

This consists of:

- Problem identification.
- Problem assessment/data collection.
- Planning interventions.
- Implementation of strategies.
- Evaluation/verification of the solution.

In essence the above model is ideally suited to support nurses in the delivery of evidence-informed practice because the skills for problem solving mirror the thinking processes associated with the evidence-informed cycle and critical appraisal.

Assessment

Within the problem-solving model, assessment is the most important element that informs evidence-based decisions. Within the Stages Theory Model of problem solving, assessment is considered as two distinct phases:

- Problem identification.
- Problem assessment.

Patient assessment is the 'deliberate and systematic collection of data to determine a client's current health status and to evaluate his present and past coping patterns' (Carpenito 1989: 45). It is a fundamental antecedent to the identification of a problem. The identification of the patient's problem is implicit within the assessment stage of problem solving. Likewise, the practising of evidence-informed nursing could begin with the identification of a clinical problem.

Data for patient problem solving or answering a research question can be collected in a variety of ways, for example:

- Interview.
- Physical examination as appropriate.
- Observation.
- Review of records and diagnostic reports.
- Collaboration with colleagues.

The purpose of collecting data within nursing is to identify the patient's past and present health status, coping patterns, responses to present problem(s) and interventions, and assessing the risk of potential problems (Carpenito 1989). Assessment is based on a model that incorporates the physical, psychological and social aspects of life. The model of assessment should reflect the nature of the clinical area or the specific type of nursing care.

The quality of the data collected during the assessment is dependent on the nurse's knowledge base, experience and philosophy. The nurse must have the ability to:

● Communicate effectively.
● Observe systematically.
● Perform a limited physical assessment.
● Differentiate between cues and inferences.
● Identify interaction patterns.
● Validate impressions.

(Carpenito 1989)

Communicating with patients includes verbal techniques, such as closed and open-ended questions with exploration of the answers, and non-verbal, such as touch, eye contact and active listening. An experienced nurse will specifically look for data based on similar situations and explore areas where a problem is suspected. A full physical examination is not performed in the UK; however, a head-to-toe inspection will be done and vital signs will be established.

The nurse then has to recognise and validate the information that has been collected. Cues are subjective statements from the patient or family and objective observations by the nurse. Inferences are the nurse's judgement or interpretations of these cues. Carpenito uses the example of a patient crying as a cue and the inference of the nurse is that he or she is sad or frightened. It is important to establish a cue as a fact, otherwise the formulation of a problem based on the nurse's interpretation of it may be erroneous and ineffective care may be given as a result. If the patient was crying because of relief or happiness, the nurse would then have intervened inappropriately.

Formulating a problem or diagnosis from data requires patterns to be identified and findings to be validated. This involves complex thinking and the use of memory to make sense of and understand the meaning of the data. Alternative explanations may be necessary at this stage until they can be ruled out. This process is described in medicine as formulating 'differential diagnosis'.

An example of this would be the nurse managing a patient who has become acutely confused following surgery. Attempts will need to be made to identify the cause of the inappropriate behaviour in order to manage it, eradicate it and prevent it occurring in the future. Possible causes would need to be considered before any treatment commences, and the doctor and nurse will discuss a number of possible causes and undertake diagnostic tests to confirm or reject them.

The above skills are essential in achieving an accurate assessment of the patient's needs. Similarly, in order to practise evidence-based nursing, the nurse needs to have the knowledge, skills and understanding to critically appraise the relevant research (Chapter 3). When referring to the above assessment of the patient's situation, the skills and systematic approaches used by the nurse are almost identical to the processes associated with practising evidence-informed nursing.

For example:

- Assess the patient's clinical situation.
- Access the appropriate research evidence.
- Critically appraise the suitability of the evidence for practice.

Decision-making

Once a problem has been formulated a decision to act should follow. There are many complex models of decision-making; however, there are two main schools of thought. These are commonly defined as the rationalist and intuitive models (Luker *et al.* 1998).

The rationalist model may be referred to as the 'scientific model' whereby an analytical approach is used to make clinical decisions. It incorporates decision analysis and is an approach utilising probability and utility theory to enable the nurse to make rational and logical decisions. The nature of the problem is identified and all available options are considered. This approach enables the nurse to make her/his knowledge and judgements explicit. This aspect is fundamental to the practice of evidence-informed care as it allows the nurse to explain and justify to the patient the reasons for the care.

The argument for using this type of decision-making approach is that the nurse can demonstrate how she/he made her/his decision to provide specific care, thereby increasing public confidence and professional accountability. However, this approach assumes that knowledge is available all of the time and that nurses have the time to demonstrate how they made their decision.

Intuitive theory states that decisions can only be made within the context of a specific situation or an individual patient. This is due to the dependence of intuitive theory on the nurse's skill to apply the findings of rational analysis to solve a specific problem and the degree of risk taking that the nurse is prepared to accept in the chaotic world of health care. This approach to decision-making is based on the nurse's tacit knowledge developed through past experiences.

To successfully practise evidence-informed nursing the unifying of both rationalist and intuitive approaches to decision-making is needed to balance the strengths and weaknesses of evidence against the clinical situation. The use of critical reflection and learning from experience is an ideal way of achieving this.

Reflective learning

If clinical reasoning can be articulated and shared with others, there is an opportunity to efficiently develop expertise in nursing. This has implications for nurses to learn to reflect and think about their work. Reflective learning is a key mechanism to encourage effective clinical decision-making and develop expertise. The mystery of how decisions are made can be understood through returning to an incident either positive or negative, or a specific patient, and reflecting on the reasoning behind the decision-making. The establishment of evidence for validating decisions and actions, either scientific (rationalist) or opinion-based (intuitive) also occurs when a discussion or the reviewing of literature is pursued and applied.

Learning through the analysis of practice experience, with either positive or negative outcomes, enables the knowledge gained or the changed perspective to be utilised during new encounters, and increases self-awareness (Johns 1995, Parker *et al.* 1995). Thinking about clinical practice and learning from everyday work has formed a large and important subject in nurse education over the last decade and is now also valued by other professions.

As previously discussed, a major influence on the decision-making process is the nurse's own philosophy and subjective inferences on the interpretation of a situation. Through the process of critical reflection, it is anticipated that personal feelings, beliefs, drives or theories that inform actions will be brought into conscious awareness, articulated and understood. Self-awareness will be increased along with the ability to make appropriate decisions and thus intervene more effectively and efficiently (Schon 1991, Parker *et al.* 1995, Newall 1992).

Boyd and Fales (1983) define reflective learning as 'the process of internally examining an issue of concern, triggered by an experience, which creates and clarifies meaning in terms of self and which results in a changed conceptual perspective'. The purpose of reflection is 'to enable the practitioner to access, understand and learn through their lived experiences and as a consequence, to take congruent action towards developing increasing effectiveness within the context of what is understood as desirable practice' (Johns 1995: 226). Argyris and Schon (1978) classified action theories as *espoused theories* (those which are learned consciously to inform action) and *theories in use* (those which are actually used in everyday practice which may be unconscious).

Reflective learning therefore aims to help nurses to understand those theories in use during their everyday work: those that inform decision-making in clinical practice. This occurs through first identifying all the factors which influenced decision-making and, secondly, making sense of them, including how they all relate to each other.

Reflecting to develop expertise

Recalling experiences is an everyday event; however, reflecting as a learning activity is a deliberate activity. In order to develop expertise, nurses need to understand what it is they do and the consequences of their actions in everyday work. Part of this process is for the nurse to understand the reasoning behind decision-making, which then informs the actions that are taken.

Mechanisms to support reflective learning therefore should focus on helping nurses to understand problems or issues they are presented with in everyday work, and articulate this to others. This will provide the necessary coaching required in the development of clinical expertise.

Reflecting to develop evidence-informed decision-making

By reflecting nurses can understand the factors, which influence decision-making and establish if there are more effective ways to intervene. Through nurses identifying problems, collecting and appraising available evidence, best practice can be established.

Reflecting in action

Reflecting in action refers to reflecting whilst 'in' the situation itself, when presented with a problem. This involves nurses paying attention to issues in front of them, and recalling their understanding of them in order to make the next decision (Schon 1991). The process is parallel to the scientific process of hypothesis testing, whereby a hypothesis is made, actions are affirmed if a positive result occurs, or negated when they do not. The ritualistic way nurses have performed in their role in the past (Walsh and Ford 1989) has led to suggestions that nurses indeed do not 'think on their feet', reflect on their actions and thereby make improvements in their practice. Nurses therefore require coaching and practice to learn how to perceive a situation, understand and recall as much existing knowledge as possible (Andrews 1996).

Reflection on action

Reflection on action involves reflecting on a situation or critical incident after it has occurred. The purpose of this is to establish why certain actions were taken, and whether they achieved what they were supposed to achieve. In other words, if something was done right and if it was the right thing to do.

Returning to an incident has its problems. It involves the recollection of events, which may be inaccurate. According to Newall (1992), events which are distressing, for example, involving a patient's excessive suffering or one's own behaviour which was in some way inappropriate or in error, may be repressed and painful to recollect. Hindsight bias may also distort the reflective process. This is where events are understood with a subjective understanding of what someone thought happened, that is, an interpretation of an event in the light of knowing the outcome (Reece Jones 1995). This is because one understands and interprets an event within a personal theory. Meaning is assigned to experience depending on past experiences and life events, as discussed earlier.

Facilitating reflective learning

Schon (1991) suggests that reflection cannot be taught, but can be coached in others in many creative ways

Journal keeping

With academic or formal learning, reflection can be coached through the writing and analysis of critical incidents, in an academic style. The process starts with the writing of a personal diary or journal, which has been described as a useful tool to examine practice (Riley-Doucet and Wilson 1997). Students are encouraged to write a diary at the end of each working day, or following an incident which has caused them unease or concern or has had a positive outcome. Walker (1985) describes how this can be cathartic and make the student feel better having expressed thoughts and feelings, 'getting them of their chest'.

The drawback in journal keeping is that it has limitations in helping to perceive an event from different perspectives, with distressing events or actions remaining unexplored because it is painful or has been repressed in order that it can be forgotten. In addition, exploration of other perspectives or ways of looking at a problem may be lost without another person's view and interpretation.

Journal keeping, however, may contribute to a greater understanding of practice and inform the writing of academic essays which solely reflect on an incident or practice event. Through the examination of the literature to justify or negate a decision to intervene in a certain way, the nurse is encouraged in the use and application of evidence to practice.

A model for reflecting

When reflecting on experience, there are a number of models available to help structure thoughts and ideas. Johns (1995) devised a model

Box 5.1 A critical incident analysis model or reflective learning framework

When describing the experience (written or verbal), the following questions can be addressed:

- What was I trying to achieve?
- Why did I respond like I did?
- What were the consequences of this for: the patient, others, myself?
- How was this person (or persons) feeling?
- How did I know that?
- How did I feel in this situation?
- What internal factors were influencing me?
- How did my actions match with my beliefs?
- What factors made me act in incongruent ways?
- What knowledge did or should have informed me?
- How does this connect with previous experiences?
- Could I handle this better in similar situations?
- What would be the consequences of alternative actions: for the patient, others, myself?
- How do I now feel about the experience?
- Can I support myself and others better as a consequence?
- Has this changed my ways of knowing?

(Source: Johns, C. (1995) Framing learning through reflection with Carper's fundamental ways of knowing in nursing, *Journal of Advanced Nursing* 22, 2, 226–34. Reprinted by kind permission of Blackwell Science Ltd, Oxford.

(Box 5.1) which can be used either to analyse a critical incident or as a framework for reflective learning within clinical supervision.

The model provides a framework for in-depth analysis of an incident, which may be rather complex for use in practice, such as a clinical supervision session. The model could, however, be adapted or shortened to accommodate the pressures of time in clinical practice.

Reflective groups

Teaching students how to reflect can also occur using the group method in academia. A number of students may meet together on a weekly basis to reflect on their practice. The process has been referred to as 'action learning', which has been adapted from an educational approach in management to encourage learning from other group members. The aim of such groups are two-fold: first, to understand and work through clinical problems in a safe setting; and, second, to learn from the experience of others (Haddock 1997).

Learning in groups, however, brings problems associated with group processes and the nature of health care. When caring for people who have health problems, nurses are often faced with issues relating to pain, suffering and/or death. This has the potential to create excessive anxiety in staff as they empathise with patients, or if they have experienced similar problems in their own life or with close family and friends (Haddock 1997). This anxiety is often difficult to deal with and is therefore repressed (forgotten) (Menzies 1970). Pressure from the group to recall such experiences may occur and create anxiety in the member. This requires an experienced facilitator to manage such pressures and anxiety.

Group dynamics may also impinge on the way group members relate to each other, for example, group members have to get to know each other in order to feel safe. This process takes time and should be considered when encouraging members to share often difficult or intimate experiences within the group. Other problems may relate to participation, either a member dominating the group or non-participation. It is important to ensure that group boundaries and ground rules are defined along with a group facilitator who is either skilled with group work or is supervised by someone who is (Haddock 1997)

When setting up such a group in clinical practice, there are many other factors to consider, such as ongoing working relationships, hierarchical or social structures which may prevent real issues being brought to the group for discussion. A more familiar group in the clinical setting would be referred to as peer supervision, which will be discussed later.

Clinical supervision

Clinical supervision has been advocated in nursing for many years, and the UKCC published a position statement in 1995 suggesting that it will play a key role in ensuring safe standards of care. Evolving from disciplines such as social work and psychotherapy, it is now considered a key mechanism in providing all clinical staff from a wide variety of professions with the necessary support, development opportunities and a method of monitoring the supervisee.

The process involves a supervisee and supervisor agreeing a period of time in which to meet and discuss issues or problems relating to the supervisee's clinical practice. Reflection on practice is therefore an essential element to help the supervisee to:

- prioritise problems for discussion during the session;
- think about the problems with a view to having a degree of insight and understanding prior to the session;
- structure the session using a reflective model such as Johns (1995), described earlie;
- be creative in overcoming any problems identified and informing an action plan from each session.

The success of using the reflective process within supervision would also be influenced by the skill of the supervisor to help the supervisee gain insight of the issues, facilitate self-awareness and provide appropriate advice in order that problems can be managed or overcome.

Clinical case presentation

The presentation of clinical cases is an established method of learning in medicine, either through bedside case discussion with a consultant and juniors or formally through presenting a patient case history which is of interest to the profession. The process requires reflecting on one's own practice and experience at all stages of the presentation, with the sharing of opinions and ideas with peers.

Presenting a clinical case can also be used within clinical supervision, providing an opportunity to examine patient assessment, decision-making, choice of intervention(s) and outcomes in greater detail.

Journal clubs

A setting which involves a group of staff meeting on a regular basis to review research evidence within their specialist area is often called a journal club/seminar. Presenting an article in depth to peers for discussion and review is a valuable exercise and opportunity to reflect on one's own practice. In addition to establishing whether the article is credible and applicable to practice, it provides an opportunity for the group members to reflect on current practice, the evidence-base that informs it and think of new ways to improve efficiency and effectiveness.

Outcomes of decision-making: Informing evidence-based nursing

One of the main challenges of evidence-based decision-making is the application of research to the individual patient or practice. Glasziou *et al.* (1998) has developed a framework to address this problem in medicine. With minor adaptations as demonstrated in Box 5.2, this could be used for nurses to link the process of decision-making and the practising of evidence-based nursing.

Box 5.2 A framework for decision-making in evidence-based nursing

Glasziou *et al.* (1998) suggest that the following questions should be asked:

● **Is my patient or this problem so different from those in the study that the results cannot be applied?**
This involves critical appraisal skills to interpret the literature and expertise to define the problem. The question could apply to any issue or problems from practice, trying to establish if the studies can give guidance in providing effective care.

● **Is the care or treatment feasible in my setting?**
This examines barriers such as geography, economics, skills and the organisation of services. Decisions to intervene which will produce 'good enough' outcomes is perhaps one of the most important influences in the success of evidence-based practice, yet is little debated. In real life, the recommendations from research reports are rarely attainable.

Box 5.2 – *continued*

- **What are the likely benefits and harms from the treatment?**
  Once the intervention required has been decided a risk assessment can be performed. The patient's/staff responsibility in the achievement of a health benefit should be made explicit, and the effects of low compliance considered.

- **How will my patients' values influence the decision?**
  Considering patients' preference is important for nursing and therapy professions where the nature of their work is based around a close relationship with patients and there is a lack of research which is prescriptive in nature. It involves the provision of necessary information in order that she/he can contribute to the decision. Each professional may need to consider how her/his own values influence a health care decision, for example, deciding when to administer analgesia to a patient.

Source: Glasziou, P. *et al.* (1998) Applying the results of trials and systematic reviews to individual patients, *Evidence-Based Medicine* 3, 6, 165–6. Reprinted by kind permission of the BMJ Publishing Group.

Using the framework in Box 5.2, the following case study demonstrates how nurses are able to make evidence-based decisions in relation to communicating news to a patient of his impending death.

Communicating bad news to patients has been the subject of many recent qualitative research studies and audit projects, both locally and nationally. Research is therefore available which has led to guidelines being produced on good practice by the King's Fund, and the Royal College of Physicians. Good practice guidelines for breaking bad news was therefore applicable to Mr James and would guide the doctor and nurse in communicating effectively to him.

Good practice involves:

- Assessing the patient and her/his family to establish their current knowledge, understanding and emotional state.
- Providing information, sensitively and optimistically, at a pace that the patient can understand.

Case study 5.1

Mr James, aged 58, had been admitted to an acute surgical ward with jaundice, abdominal pain, vomiting and a bowel obstruction. Following a number of investigations and a laparotomy, it was established that he had primary bowel cancer with multiple secondary deposits in the abdomen including extensive liver involvement. His prognosis was very poor with an estimated survival of 9–12 months. He now needed to have this information communicated to him and his family.

- Ensuring the patient has comfort, privacy and time to express emotion and ask questions.

When establishing if this is feasible for Mr James, consideration would be given to ensuring the nurse and doctor have experience and adequate skills in giving bad news. This would involve having knowledge of Mr James and his family's emotional and physical state, estimating if possible the level and detail of information he may want to hear, and providing it in a sensitive manner.

Providing privacy for Mr James will depend on having a private room to sit in away from the noisy ward, and his physical state, that is, for him to be able to leave his bed. Timing of giving the bad news may also depend on his psychological state and conscious level; for example, if he is receiving regular opioids, he would not be able to understand what is being said.

When considering the benefit and harm of giving bad news, the nurse would consider whether giving the prognosis in great detail would distress Mr James or be beneficial to him in coming to terms with his illness. A relative may be judged to be emotionally unstable, which may have a detrimental effect on how Mr James may deal with the information. The nurse may decide to discuss with the doctor how the relative could be told.

The values of the patient, doctor and nurse would influence how the information was given and received. Mr James may have strong religious beliefs about life after death, which may help to reduce his distress. His values on his own life will effect his response and decision for further treatment and care, and the nurse should try to be sensitive to these when information is given.

The values of the nurse and doctor may affect the way that information is given. If, for example, the nurse is excessively fearful of her/his own death, then information may be given in an excessively optimistic manner, perhaps with too much reassurance that all will be well, essentially denying that the patient is not really approaching premature death. This would be to protect the nurse from experiencing her own distress, rather than considering the needs of the patient.

Although information should be provided with optimism, in that all that is possible will be done to increase the patients survival time, a balance has to be made with the statistical facts of survival time to ensure the patient is not led into believing his illness does not exist.

Clinical guidelines

Following the appraisal of the evidence, the development of clinical guidelines may follow, particularly for those cases that are more common and clear criteria can be developed to reduce variation in practice.

For more information, read Chapter 4 and the section subtitled 'Integrated care pathways'.

Conclusion

An important challenge for nurses is coaching the development of clinical expertise along with the evidence-base and rationale behind decision-making. To assist nurses in the articulation of the rationale informing decisions, the publication of evidence-informed case studies or reports on difficult decisions or interesting patients in nursing would be of benefit. Although there has been an increase in the publication of critical incident analysis and narratives from nursing practice, nurses should be encouraged to describe cases and how problems were identified, with supporting literature to justify decisions.

Nurses require opportunities to reflect on their practice, locate and read available evidence to critically appraise an issue or topic identified within their practice. This will contribute to improving the services provided within a ward or department through the development of critically appraised topics relevant to the area of practice. Research evidence, professional bodies and interest groups may have already developed clinical guidelines in some areas. However, appraisal of the research literature at ward or department level can be used to develop local evidence-based guidelines for practice.

This will contribute to the nurse's own professional development and learning by working through the process of evidence-informed decision-making, providing evidence-informed care and identifying standards/guidelines to audit the effectiveness of nursing practice. Since clinical guidelines require updating as new research is produced, reviewing them or producing new ones will provide the ward, department or specialist area an opportunity to reduce the risks of harming patients and demonstrate the use of evidence-informed practice.

Summary of key points

- Reflective practice is an essential component of evidence-informed practice.
- Reflection in action enables the nurse to utilise their current knowledge of evidence in the immediate decision-making process when providing nursing care.
- Reflection on action enables the nurse to define and respond to a clinical situation after the event and evaluate the effectiveness of their action(s).
- Reflection in or on positive or negative experiences stimulates nurses to question the evidence underpinning their practice.
- There are various strategies nurses can use to facilitate reflective practice.

Recommended reading

Argyris, C. and Schon, D. (1978) *Theory in Practice: Increasing Professional Effectiveness* Massachusetts, Addison Wesley Johns, C. (1995) The value of reflective practice for nursing, *Journal of Clinical Nursing* 4, 23–30

References

Andrews, M. (1996) Using reflection to develop clinical expertise, *British Journal of Nursing* 5, 8, 508–13.

Argyris, C. and Schon D. (1978) *Theory in Practice: Increasing Professional Effectiveness* Massachusetts, Addison Wesley.

Benner, P. (1984) *From Novice to Expert: Excellence and Power in Clinical Nursing Practice* California, Addison Wesley.

Boyd, E.M. and Fales, A.W. (1983) Reflective learning: Key to learning from experience, *Journal of Human Psychology* 23, 2, 99–117.

Carpenito, L.J. (1989) *Nursing Diagnosis: Application to Clinical Practice*, 3rd Ed Philadelphia, J.B. Lippincott Company.

Ford, M. and Walsh, P. (1989) *Nursing Rituals: Research And Rational Actions* Oxford, Butterworth Heinemann.

Glasziou, P., Guyatt, G.H., Dans, A.L., Dans, L.F., Straus, S. and Sackett, D. L. (1998) Applying the results of trials and systematic reviews to individual patients, *Evidence-Based Medicine* 3, 6, 165–6.

Haddock, J. (1997) Reflection in groups: Contextual and theoretical considerations within nurse education and practice, *Nurse Education Today* 17, 381–5.

Haynes, B., Sackett, D., Gray, J.M., Cook, D. and Guyatt, G. (1996). Transferring evidence from research into practice: 1. The role of clinical care research evidence in clinical decisions, *Evidence Based Medicine* Nov/Dec, 196–7.

Hurst, K., Dean, A. and Trickey, S. (1991) The recognition and non-recognition of problem-solving stages in nursing practice, *Journal of Advanced Nursing* 16, 1444–55.

Johns, C. (1995) The value of reflective practice for nursing, *Journal of Clinical Nursing* 4, 23–30.

Luker, K.A., Hogg, C., Austin, L., Ferguson, B. and Smith, K. (1998). Decision-making: The context of nurse prescribing, *Journal of Advanced Nursing* 27, 657–65.

Menzies, I.E.P. (1970) *The Functioning of Social Systems as a Defence Against Anxiety* London, Tavistock Publications.

Newall, R. (1992) Anxiety, accuracy and reflection: The limits of professional development, *Journal of Advanced Nursing* 17, 1326–33

Parker, D.L., Webb, J. and D'Souza, B. (1995) The value of critical incident analysis as an educational tool and in relationship to experiential learning, *Nurse Education Today* 15, 111–16.

Polanyi, M. (1958) *Personal Knowledge* London, Routledge and Kegan Paul.

Reece Jones, P. (1995) Hindsight bias in reflective practice: An empirical investigation, *Journal of Advanced Nursing* 21, 783–8.

Riley-Doucet, C. and Wilson, S. (1997) A three-step method of self-reflection using reflective journal writing, *Journal of Advanced Nursing* 25, 964–8.

Royal College of Physicians (1997) *Improving Communication between Doctors and Patients* London, Royal College of Physicians.

Schon, D. (1991) *The Reflective Practitioner*, 2nd edn, San Francisco, Jossey Bass.

Walker, D. (1985) Ch 3, Writing and reflection. In Boud D., Keogh, R. and Walker, D. (eds) *Reflection: Turning Experience into Learning* London, Kogan Page.

Walsh, M. and Ford, P. (1989) *Nursing Rituals: Research and Rational Actions* Oxford, Heinemann Nursing.

Chapter 6
Evidence into practice

Louise Brereton

Introduction

The importance of evidence-informed practice and the benefits of research for clinical practice have been established previously in Chapters 1 and 4 of this book. Additionally Chapters 2 and 3 have helped you to develop some understanding of what research is, how information (data) is collected and how to critically review research papers. Chapter 5 highlighted the importance of reflection on practice.

This chapter builds on the knowledge and skills that you have already gained by inviting you to reflect on your practice and to critically consider the evidence on which that practice is based. This is a practical chapter that uses a case study approach to illustrate how the skills and knowledge you will have developed from the previous chapters can assist you in practising evidence-informed nursing associated with promoting 'sleep'. This is achieved by the application of the evidence-informed nursing cycle identified in Chapter 1, Figure 1.1. The example by-passes the research awareness phase because we hope that, through reading and reflecting upon Chapter 2, you will be more confident with research and where it fits with practising evidence-informed nursing.

Evidence into practice: Sleep

To demonstrate how evidence-informed nursing could assist with either resolving clinical problems and/or developing innovations in clinical practice the following case study will be used.

Case study 6.1

Joe Smith is a 72-year-old gentleman who was admitted to hospital for a hip replacement. He is now completing his rehabilitation, but staff are concerned that Joe is not sleeping at night, reporting 'poor night's sleep' in the nursing notes. Joe often doesn't go to sleep until the early hours of the morning and, despite this, he wakes early too. It is suggested that the doctor is asked to prescribe some night sedation for Joe. However, Joe refuses to take the night sedation when it is offered, despite efforts by the staff to persuade him to do so. Joe explains that he never goes to bed until midnight and rises at about 5am every morning. He works for long hours in his garden or greenhouses when he is at home, but has been bored and cannot sleep in hospital because he has nothing to do.

How can evidence assist the nurses in resolving the above clinical problem?

Step 1: Reflecting on the issues

A number of issues arise from Case study 6.1. There appears to have been no reference to the nursing assessment of Joe's normal sleeping pattern, nor have his views about his sleeping pattern been documented in the nursing notes. Staff have resorted to the use of night sedation without apparently discussing this with Joe or considering alternative actions. Clearly, there is a need to base care on a problem-solving approach, rather than merely adopting actions that may be inappropriate to the individual patient's needs. However, whilst Walsh and Ford (1989) suggest that the use of a problem solving approach may avoid ritualistic care, Cohen and Mannion (1985) suggest that even when nurses use this approach, the knowledge applied is often based on rituals and tradition. We will return to the use of rituals and traditions in nursing later in this chapter. While Case study 6.1 reflects some of the issues reported in the nursing literature about promoting sleep, it is useful to reflect on your own experience.

Activity 6.1 Reflect on your own experience of nursing a patient who had problems sleeping

Use a pen and paper to complete the rest of this exercise. Divide the page into 3 columns entitled: (a) assessment, (b) goals and intervention, and (c) evidence used. Now complete each column by answering the following questions:

Column a – What assessment was completed of the patient's problem and how was it completed?

Column b – What goals and nursing actions were planned to promote sleep?

Column c – What evidence supports each of the nursing actions that were planned? (i.e. How do you know that what you do works?)

Keep the exercise that you have just completed as we will re-examine this once we have considered some of the literature available about sleep problems for hospitalised patients.

Step 2: The need to identify and gather the evidence

To identify the most up-to-date information, a literature search needs to be completed

Finding the evidence

Clearly, if you want to find research to implement into practice, you will need to develop effective literature searching skills. However, knowing where to find the evidence and making research findings available to nurses will not alone effect a change in practice (NHS Centre for Reviews and Dissemination 1999). With regard to the literature and literature searching, a number of initiatives have been developed to promote research utilisation in practice (see Box 6.1).

Box 6.1 Sources to aid retrieval of research literature

- *Summary of research findings*
  - Systematic reviews and Meta Analysis and clinical guidelines/integrated care pathways.
- *Dissemination and Implementation:*
  - Clinical Effectiveness in *Nursing Quarterly Journal* focusing on the effectiveness of clinical interventions.
  - Evidence-based *Nursing Quarterly Journal* that identifies and appraises high quality clinical related research.
  - Centre for Evidence-Based Nursing: <http://www.york.ac.uk/depts/hstd/centres/evidence/ev-intra.htm>
  - Dynamic Quality Improvement Network RCN Program: <http://www.rcn.org.uk/services/practice/quality/quality.htm#dqi>
  - MIDIRS (Midwives Information and Resource Services: <http://www.midirs.org>
- *Electronic databases:*
  - British Nursing Index – CD Rom Cumulative Index to Nursing and Allied health literature: database covers all aspects of nursing and allied health disciplines.

Box 6.1 – *continued*

- ENB Health Care Database – references and abstracts from all the 80 UK journals since 1985: <http://www.enb.org.uk/hcd.htm>
- Nursing and Health Care Research on the Web: <http://www.shef.ac.uk/-nhron>

Focusing on the research relating to the activity of living associated with sleep may assist in highlighting the complex nature of using research in practice. In this case study example relating to sleep as an activity of daily living, the Cochran database was searched using the keyword 'sleep'. Although a vast amount of research was found relating to sleep, this did not focus on nursing patients suffering from sleeplessness and was therefore of no use. Subsequently, the computer databases MEDLINE and CINAHL were searched again using the keyword 'Sleep', which identified a wealth of information about the broader aspects of sleep. This search revealed an enormous amount of literature that would have been unrealistic and impractical to review (time and resources). So what do you do in this situation?

In clinical practice you may find that there is too much or too little or no research directly related to the area of care you are investigating. Therefore, you may need to focus or explore related issues and consider if the principles of evidence from these related issues are of value to your specific clinical interest. For example, in light of the initial literature search a change in the search strategy was required to limit the amount of information to the topic under review. For example, articles can be limited by date, research papers only, abstracts available and/or by a combined search. In this case a combined search was applied using the key words 'sleep' and 'nursing care'. Box 6.2 shows the stages of this literature search.

When referring back to Case study 6.1 and the exercise identified in Step 1, a 'broad brush' approach (Burnard 1993) to literature searching was initially used to identify 30 articles. Following this an 'incremental search' (Burnard 1993) was used to find a further 10 articles from the references of those initially retrieved.

Box 6.2 Literature search

a   Key word search: 'sleep' and 'nursing care'
b   Databases used: CINAHL, MEDLINE
c   Criteria for inclusion/exclusion of the studies: abstracts, research studies, literature reviews. English language. Last 15 years.
d   Retrieval of articles was limited to local holdings. A total of 30 articles were initially retrieved.
e   The literature retrieved was categorised into 13 literature reviews and 17 research papers. The research formed two broad groups of evidence:

Qualitative studies

One research paper used an exclusively qualitative approach to examine factors affecting patients' sleep. Some research combined qualitative and quantitative approaches. The qualitative aspects of research seemed to focus on sleep quality, although this was measured using a structured questionnaire and reported in a quantitative fashion.

Quantitative studies

The majority of the research found was quantitative. The strength of evidence varied – one paper used a Randomised Controlled Trial (RCT) design; five used experimental or quasi-experimental designs aimed at testing interventions; and the remaining ten were descriptive surveys examining factors affecting sleep, especially noise and the quality of sleep.

f   The literature retrieved could be categorised into:
  – Broad aspects: purpose of sleep; sleep problems; factors influencing sleep; and nursing interventions
  – Themes: insomnia, sleep deprivation in hospital; reasons for sleeplessness in hospital; assessment of sleep; promoting sleep; medication and other interventions.

Having established the existence of evidence and where to obtain the information on sleep, how do you know what is the best sources of evidence to support you in advancing this area of practice?

Sources and strength of evidence on which to base care

Having obtained all the evidence, the skills of critical appraisal as described in Chapter 3 need to be applied to the literature. Muir Gray (1997) suggests a hierarchy of the type and strength of evidence on which practice can be based (see Chapter 1). The strength of evidence is rated I–VI, with the best evidence being produced by experimental research in which sources of bias and confounding variables (factors which may influence the results) are controlled.

There is clearly an emphasis on evidence from quantitative research to support practice and debate exists regarding the appropriateness of this because it appears to overlook the value of qualitative studies. Quantitative research tests theory (Depoy and Gitlin 1994) in order to provide knowledge on which to base care. Concerns have been expressed that if, as DiCenso and Cullum (1998) suggest, the best evidence is considered to be developed from RCTs, then nursing will be disadvantaged because the methodology would not motivate nurses and the criteria for such research trials would be difficult to adhere to (Reagan 1998). Furthermore, Freak (1995) highlights that concern has been expressed about the 'statistical standard' of many published RCTs. Qualitative research is used to develop theory, insight and understanding (Depoy and Gitlin 1994) and therefore plays an essential role in developing the knowledge on which nursing care can be based. Lloyd-Smith (1996) points out that qualitative research can provide knowledge that quantitative research cannot. Perhaps the most appropriate stance is to value each type of research for what it has to offer, rather than adopt a polarised view of which is the best.

Having identified and 'themed' the literature, the next step is to critically appraise it. To ensure that you review the literature effectively, it is essential that you are confident to critically appraise the information. To help you achieve this, read Chapter 3 on developing critical appraisal skills.

Step 3: Reviewing the evidence from the literature search

Having obtained all the evidence, the skills of critical appraisal as described in Chapter 3 need to be applied to the literature. Following critical appraisal of the literature, the findings need to be analysed for their implications to the clinical situation in question. To achieve this it may be helpful to work from the broad to the specific. For example: What is sleep? Why do individuals need sleep? What causes sleeplessness? How can nurses promote sleep? This approach is illustrated below in relation to Case study 6.1.

Broad aspects of the literature review

The essential function of sleep has not yet been established (Hodgson 1991, Dorociak 1990, Duxbury 1994a), although much research suggests that sleep deprivation is detrimental to an individual's physical and psychological well-being (Closs 1988, Shapiro and Flanigan 1993, Southwell and Wistow 1995b). A wealth of evidence indicates that patients suffer from sleep deprivation in hospital (King Edward's Hospital Fund for London 1960, Carter 1985, Hill 1989, Ward 1992, Southwell and Wistow 1995b, Marcus 1995, Mantle 1996), with suggestions that as many as 20–30 per cent of hospital patients are affected (Baldwin and Hopcroft 1987). Ensuring that patients have adequate sleep and rest in hospital are important nursing goals to promote patient recovery (Wilkie 1990, Brugne 1994, Southwell and Whistow 1995a). You will probably have nursed several patients who have had difficulty sleeping whilst they were in hospital.

The specific aspects of the literature review

Insomnia Investigators and subjects use many different definitions and interpretations for the term insomnia (Duxbury 1994b). Although insomnia may be used simply to refer to dissatisfaction with sleep (Oswald and Adam 1983), as many as 88 types of sleeping disorders have been reported (Becker and Jamieson 1992). Given the number and types of insomnia, for the purposes of this chapter insomnia will simply refer to sleeplessness.

Sleep deprivation in hospital   The need for sleep increases during illness and stress (Adam and Oswald 1984, Southwell and Wistow 1995b). Despite this, Stead (1984) identified that night nurses implemented set sleeping patterns, including waking times, and continued unnecessary observations on patients throughout the night that resulted in sleep deprivation. Much of the literature regarding sleep deprivation in hospital has focused on elderly patients, probably because sleep efficiency declines with age (George 1985, Kearnes 1989, Matthews *et al.* 1996) and one-third of all prescriptions for this age group are for hypnotics (Damle 1989, Duxbury 1994b).

Reasons for sleeplessness in hospital   Dunwell (1995) categorised the reasons under four themes, physical, psychological, environmental and lifestyle factors. There are many possible reasons why patients suffer from insomnia whilst they are in hospital, but the most widely recognised cause is noise (Closs 1988, Dias 1992, Haddock 1994, Southwell and Wistow 1995b) which is a problem particularly in high dependency areas such as intensive and coronary care units (Topf *et al.* 1996).

Assessing patients' sleep   Analysis of the literature suggests that support exists for a number of the factors identified by Dunwell, and several writers have emphasised the role of nurses as essential in promoting sleep (Wilkie 1990, Burton 1992, Dias 1992, Southwell and Wistow 1995a). The notion that insomnia refers to an individual's dissatisfaction with their sleep has important implications for the assessment of sleep. Clearly, this suggests that there needs to be a subjective element to the assessment of sleep for patients in hospital. There has been support for the assessment of a patient's normal sleep routine (Dootson 1990) as well as assessment of any problems experienced (Edell-Gustafsson *et al.* 1994, Dunwell 1995, Southwell and Wistow 1995b). Bowman (1997) appears to have addressed this issue in her American study of elderly patients following planned or emergency orthopaedic hip surgery. The study investigated 43 patients' satisfaction with sleep, using a 7-point likert scale, ranging from 1, extremely poorly, to 7, extremely well. The findings suggest that sleep satisfaction was markedly poorer in patients who suffered delirium, which Bowman suggests is a common phenomenon following orthopaedic surgery.

Southwell and Wistow (1995b) also appear to have addressed this issue in their British survey of patients' perceptions of sleep in three hospitals in different types of geographical areas. The authors developed two questionnaires to survey patient and staff views. Data were collected from respondents (454 patients and 218 staff) in a variety of ward areas including general medicine, surgery, elderly and acute psychiatry. The patient questionnaire collected a range of data, including information about sleep and disturbances and overall satisfaction. The findings suggest that half of the patients surveyed did not get as much sleep as they needed. Interestingly, although staff recognised that patients did not get as much sleep as they needed, they did not attribute this to their own behaviour. This study did not investigate the documentation of patients' sleep problems by nurses, which may be important if action is to be taken to address the problem. However, a number of writers have reported that nurses fail to document information about patients' sleep in the nursing records (Kemp 1984, Southwell and Wistow 1995a and b). The problem is not restricted to the UK. Edell-Gustafsson *et al.* (1994) evaluated patient records with regard to nurses' documentation of sleep in the first four post-operative days for 80 male patients undergoing coronary artery by-pass surgery in Sweden.

The study involved retrospective analysis of data collected from the nursing notes about both the quantity and quality of sleep. The writers reported that there were few notes about either the duration or quality of sleep. Additionally, the accuracy of the documentation was questioned as the records were based on short, random observations of the patients. As such, the authors suggest that a more structured description is needed of patients' sleep. Clearly, a limitation of this Swedish study is that it ignores the patients' subjective view of sleep, which is important.

Promoting sleep The information provided about sleep and the assessment of sleep may already enable you to reflect on Activity 6.1 that you completed earlier. You should be able to consider the appropriateness of your suggested patient assessment (Column a) and the interventions in your care plan (Column b). Before examining your care plan further, attention needs to be given to the actions that nurses can take to promote sleep.

Over-reliance on medication   Several writers have suggested that ritualistic care is implemented when patients experience problems sleeping in hospital (Ogilvie 1980, Webster and Thompson 1986). The most common approach to dealing with insomnia is the administration of medication (Halfens *et al.* 1991) and there have even been unsubstantiated suggestions that nurses request night sedation for patients to relieve their own frustrations rather than to help patients to sleep (Webster and Thompson 1986)! Much of the available research relates to the effectiveness of medication and is aimed primarily at a medical or pharmacology audience, perhaps reflecting the use of medication to deal with sleep problems. Nurses need to consider this information as it has been suggested that they influence junior doctors in prescribing these drugs (Duxbury 1994a) and make decisions about administering them (Halfens *et al.* 1991). Given that concerns have been expressed regarding the addictive effect (MacGregor and Lannigan 1992) and over pre-scription of night sedation (Burton 1992), along with evidence suggesting that long-term use of such medication is ineffective (Burton 1992), nurses need to consider alternative interventions (Kearnes 1989). This is particularly important in light of Halfens *et al.*'s (1991) study which found that patients who used sleep med-ication in hospital for a period of at least five days were more likely to use this on returning home than patients who did not take such medication in hospital.

Some evidence exists to suggest that most nurses believe that medication should not be used until other options have been con-sidered (Halfens *et al.* 1991). Brugne (1994) suggests that education is an essential part of the nurse's role to reduce the reliance that many individuals have on night sedation, a view supported by Childs-Clarke (1990).

Clearly, nurses will only be able to achieve this if they are willing to adopt other measures themselves. Duxbury (1994c) agrees that nursing interventions based on individualised patient assessments and preferences need to be planned rather than resorting immedi-ately to the administration of 'prn sedation'. However, despite recognition of the importance of the nurse's role in promoting sleep, there has been little research into the effectiveness of other measures (Bowman 1997).

Other interventions With reference to the factors affecting patients' ability to sleep in hospital, nurses can use a number of simple interventions to promote sleep for patients. Environmental factors, particularly noise from nurses talking, other patients and treatments are major causes of sleep disturbance for patients (Dias 1992, Marcus 1995, Southwell and Wistow 1995b, Topf *et al.* 1996). Many suggestions have been put forward about ways in which noise can be reduced on the ward, including patients using earplugs (Dias 1992). Haddock (1994) aimed to find out if the quantity and quality of patient's sleep improved when earplugs were worn compared to the previous night's sleep and other patients who did not wear ear plugs. Eighteen patients were 'paired' into two groups, those wearing earplugs and those not wearing earplugs. All patients completed a questionnaire about the quantity and quality of their sleep in hospital over three nights. The results suggest that noise was a major factor causing sleep deprivation in hospital. Earplugs were acceptable to patients, with 66 per cent (six patients) reporting improved quality and quantity of sleep when wearing them. Clearly, this small-scale study requires replication to establish the effectiveness of earplugs in promoting sleep for patients in hospital.

Sleep deprivation results from physiological factors such as pain and discomfort, and psychological factors such as anxiety (Edell-Gustafsson *et al.* 1994, Dunwell 1995, Marcus 1995, Clark *et al.* 1995, Bowman 1997). Southwell and Wistow's (1995b) survey established that discomfort, worry and pain were reported as major factors causing sleeplessness by the patients sampled. Similarly, Bowman's (1996) survey found that pain, fear and worry were reported by more patients who underwent unplanned emergency surgery for hip replacement than for patients whose surgery had been planned. Furthermore, pain scores were higher and sleep satisfaction was poorer amongst patients who suffered delirium post-operatively. The implications of these studies are clear. Nurses need to provide adequate pain relief at night (Wilkie 1990), although Closs (1988) reported that patients were less likely to receive pain relief at night. The relationship between pain experience and anxiety has long been established (Hayward 1975). Clearly, nurses need to use effective communication strategies to allay patients' fears and anxiety and also assist in reducing their pain experience.

Brugne (1994) suggests that, along with reducing noise to a minimum, establishing bedtime routines and using complementary therapies to induce sleep are all strategies that the nurse can adopt to promote sleep. Hudson (1994) briefly reports on a trial testing the benefits of lavender oil to aid relaxation in elderly patients, a group known to suffer from insomnia and poor quality sleep. Although the sample was very small, data were collected over a period of 102 patient nights and 103 patient days. The findings suggest that 84 per cent of the elderly people sampled reported sleeping well and 70 per cent had alert active days when lavender oil was used to promote sleep. During the control period, only 64 per cent reported that they had slept well, with 15 per cent having woken or slept poorly. Similarly, Cannard (1995) reported an increase from 80 per cent to 97 per cent in the number of older patients stating that they had slept well following the introduction of aromatherapy on a nursing development unit. However, the sample size was also small, thus limiting the generalisability of the findings.

Step 4: Acting on the findings from the reviewed evidence

It would be useful here to re-examine your responses to Activity 6.1 that you completed at the start of this chapter.

When referring back to Case study 6.1 and Activity 6.1, it is clear that promoting sleep involves more than just the administration of night sedation. To promote optimal sleep for our patients requires a thorough assessment of the individual's normal sleep patterns and how this has been affected by their current admission into hospital and as a direct result of their illness/disease. It requires more than just noting 'no problems' in the activities of daily living column as outlined in Activity 6.1 Feedback (see pages 112–13).

In particular, Column c asked you to identify the evidence you used to promote sleep for your patients. In the light of the literature obtained and reviewed here, is there a need for you to implement changes in practice based on this evidence? It is clear from the literature that there are multiple reasons why patients find it difficult to sleep in hospital, reinforcing the need for an individualised nursing assessment of this specific activity of living. Historically, medication has been an intervention used to promote sleep. However, other interventions have been highlighted that could also be used in promoting sleep.

Chapter 7 describes in detail how implementing evidence into your practice can be successfully achieved. For completeness of this chapter some of the issues related to implementing evidence into practice are highlighted to enable you to have some insight into the final step of implementing evidence into your own practice and in resolving Case study 6.1.

The limitations of research in providing evidence for practice

Whilst research can produce the strongest evidence on which to base practice, it is not possible to base all nursing practice on research because not all research is directly usable in practice (Tierney 1987, McDonnell 1998). Some aspects of nursing are not easily researched, for example areas that pose ethical problems. Other research aims to develop research tools and is therefore primarily of methodological use (Rodgers 1994). Furthermore, as Kitson (1997) highlights, research is relatively new to nursing, and there is still a need to complete much descriptive and observational work. Given the importance that has been afforded to research as evidence, it would seem almost unthinkable that, where indicated, the available research isn't used in practice. However, traditions and rituals seem to dominate much nursing practice.

Traditions and rituals governing nursing practice

Much nursing care is based on tradition and rituals rather than research evidence (Walsh and Ford 1989, DOH 1991). Walsh and Ford (1989) describe a number of nursing practices that are based on myths and rituals, despite the fact that research evidence exists to the contrary, with some practice being continued despite evidence that it was harmful to patients! Indeed, many writers have

Activity 6.1 Feedback

Reflections on practice

Use the information that you documented here to consider the appropriateness of the assessment, goals and interventions that you have listed below. Does the information in Columns a and b reflect the patient's individual concerns and preferences?

Column a

Assessment

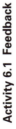

- Individual norms – their routine; the amount of sleep needed and quality of sleep.
- What problems is the patient experiencing in hospital? Document the nature, extent and effects of these problems.
- How satisfied is the patient with the quality of sleep they are getting in hospital?

Column b

Goals and interventions

- Attempt to replicate the patient's normal sleep pattern if possible and bear in mind the need for increased sleep at times of illness.
- Reduce factors that the patient identifies as causing sleeplessness – for example, increase comfort; reduce pain, fear and anxiety; reduce noise from staff,

Column c

Evidence

- Overall the evidence-base for the interventions identified in Column b is limited because there is little Type I evidence available on which to plan the patient's care. The majority of the literature used as evidence is limited by the small, convenience samples used in the studies reviewed. This means that other patients and treatments.

- Use aids such as earplugs to promote sleep.
- Employ alternative therapies such as relaxation, lavender oils and aromatherapy to promote sleep.
- Educate regarding the problems associated with night sedation.
- Administer prescribed night sedation.
- Patients to continually reassess/evaluate their sleep satisfaction using a simple structured questionnaire.
- Document information about the quantity and quality of the patient's sleep in the nursing notes.

the results are limited in their generalisability and practice developments should be implemented cautiously.

identified nurses' failure to implement research findings in practice (Hunt 1981, Brett 1989, Armitage 1990, MacGuire 1990, DOH 1991, Hunter and Pollitt 1992). More recently, DiCenso and Cullum (1998) also acknowledge this and suggest that the situation is not unique to nursing. If changes are to be made, we need to understand why nursing care is often based on tradition rather than research evidence.

Figure 6.1 illustrates the factors influencing research utilisation by nurses in practice.

A number of themes emerge from the illustration, including factors related to the culture of nursing, the attitude of the nurse, organisational influences and the support and leadership avail-

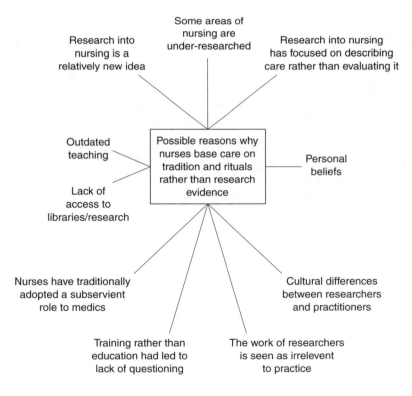

Figure 6.1 Factors influencing research utilisation by nurses.

able. Several writers have identified all of these themes as important influences affecting research utilisation in practice (Closs and Cheater 1994, Rodgers 1994, Crow *et al.* 1997, Kitson 1997, Reagan 1998).

There needs to be a positive research culture, interest from the potential nurse users of research and, finally, wide-ranging support from peers, managers and the government. The Department of Health (1993) suggests that it is the impact of research on practice which is most important. As such, there is a need to further explore these influences on research utilisation.

Culture can be defined as commonly held beliefs, attitudes and values that exist in organisations, which Closs and Cheater (1994) suggest are based on historical factors and relationships. The nursing culture will be unique to each ward or unit and will be influenced by a number of factors which exist both within and externally to the organisation, many of which are very resistant to change (Walsh and Ford 1989). Walsh (1997) suggests that a profound change in NHS culture is needed to assist research utilisation. He explains that the culture is dominated by heavy workloads, continual change, threats of staff reductions and traditional boundaries of professional practice, all of which are major hindrances. Crow *et al.* (1997) report on five focus groups involving lecturers with a specific responsibility for the development of research. Participants in all groups highlighted that tensions exist between the cultures of the NHS and higher education. The report seems to include reference to many of the issues identified by Walsh (1997) as influencing the research culture. The recent integration of nursing and midwifery into higher education was recognised as a major cultural influence. This move has served to reinforce the urgency of developing research skills and valuing time spent on research in light of the Research Assessment Exercise (RAE), which provides funding councils with information to assist in resource allocation. There was also recognition of the influence of multi-disciplinary working on the choice of research methodologies used in research or viewed as evidence because of the apparent dominance of medicine. McMahon (1997) reinforces all of these suggestions, but also acknowledges 'the absence of a nursing voice' in the Research and Development strategy.

McMahon (1996) emphasises the need for strong academic leadership and organisational support if Research and Development are to become established in the healthcare culture. Closs and Cheater (1994) suggest that the culture also needs to value ideas, innovations and research as essential prerequisites to implementing research findings in practice. Walsh (1997) advocates that nursing research needs to 'be done by some, facilitated by others and implemented by all'. However, Hunt (1981) suggested that nurses lacked the skills to apply research in practice. Whilst this may have been the case almost two decades ago, there is a danger that this will become a self-fulfilling prophecy unless a positive attitude is adopted to nurses' ability to implement research in practice by both the potential users of research and those best placed to support them in achieving this.

Step 5: Evaluation

Evaluation is a key part of the evidence-informed cycle and one which can all too easily be overlooked following the implementation of an innovation. The method of evaluation should be considered at the beginning of the evidence-informed process. Following acknowledgment of the problem, in this case sleeplessness, an assessment of the problem should be documented, if possible using a valid, reliable, systematic tool or, where this is not available, a detailed description of the problem. Following implementation of the evidence, the assessment should be repeated and the findings compared to the original assessment to evaluate if there has been any effect. For example, how long did the patient sleep before and after the intervention, how did the patient feel about their sleep pattern before and after, etc. . . . Without evaluation the process of evidence-informed practice is at risk of exchanging old rituals for new and the effectiveness of the nursing intervention remains unknown and questionable.

Conclusion

Evidence-informed nursing relies, in part, on research utilisation in practice. There is an emphasis on quantitative research to provide the best evidence on which to base practice and debate exists as to the appropriateness of this given the humanistic nature of nursing. The role of qualitative research in informing practice needs to be considered since this provides useful knowledge for practitioners. However, it would appear that nursing practice is often governed by tradition. This is hardly surprising since reference to the literature about sleep has revealed that nursing research exists, although it is often small scale. Research utilisation in practice has been identified as a complex issue. Although much research exists about the barriers to research utilisation (see Chapter 7), little appears to concentrate on the processes of implementing research into the clinical setting. Government directives have led to the development of R&D infrastructures. This chapter has demonstrated how the evidence-informed process can be used to implement evidence-based practice. However, there is now a need to identify how nurses can work in partnerships to further realise the potential of research to aid new or to evaluate established nursing practices.

Summary of key points

- To ensure that evidence-informed practice exists, it is essential that the starting point of this process be about establishing the reasons for reviewing the practice.
- Time invested in accessing a wide range of data sources to inform the literature review is time well spent.
- Critically reviewing the literature and identifying the current evidence-base to inform the practice under review might mean exploring issues beyond those initially anticipated.
- It is important to emphasis that changing practice is time consuming and requires focused commitment if the change is be successfully made in practice.

Recommended reading

Bowman, A.M. (1997) Sleep satisfaction, perceived pain and acute confusion in elderly clients undergoing orthopaedic procedures, *Journal of Advanced Nursing* 26, 550–64

Childs-Clarke, A. (1990) Stimulus control techniques for sleep onset insomnia, *Nursing Times* 86, 35, 52–3

MacGuire, J. (1990) Putting nursing research findings into practice: Research utilisation as an aspect of the management of change, *Journal of Advanced Nursing* 15, 614–20

Southwell, M. and Wistow, G. (1995a) Sleep in hospitals at night: Are patients' needs being met? *Journal of Advanced Nursing* 21, 1101–9

References

Adam, K. and Oswald, I. (1984) Sleep helps healing, *British Medical Journal* 289, 1400–1.

Armitage, S. (1990) Research utilisation in practice. *Nurse Education Today* 10, 1, 10–15.

Baldwin, D. and Hopcroft, K. (1987) *A Handbook for Housemen* London, Blackwell Scientific Publications.

Becker, P.M. and Jamieson, A.O. (1992) Common sleep disorders in the elderly. Diagnosis and treatment, *Geriatrics* 47, 3, 41–52.

Bowman, A.M. (1997) Sleep satisfaction, perceived pain and acute confusion in elderly clients undergoing orthopaedic procedures. *Journal of Advanced Nursing* 26, 550–64.

Brett, J.L.L. (1989) Use of nursing practice research findings, *Nursing Research* 36, 6, 344–9.

Brugne, J.-F. (1994) Sleep, wakefulness and the nurse, *British Journal of Nursing* 3, 2, 68–71.

Burnard, P. (1993) Facilities for searching the literature and storing references, *Nurse Researcher* 1, 1, 56–63.

Burton, E. (1992) Something to help you sleep? *Nursing Times* 88, 8, 52–4

Cannard, G. (1995) On the scent of a good night's sleep, *Nursing Standard* 9, 34, 21.

Carter, D. (1985) Sleepless nights: In need of a good night's sleep, *Nursing Times* 81, 46, 24–6.

Childs-Clarke, A. (1990) Stimulus control techniques for sleep onset insomnia, *Nursing Times* 86, 35, 52–3.

Clark, A.J., Flowers, J., Boots, L. and Shettar, S. (1995) Sleep disturbance in mid-life women, *Journal of Advanced Nursing* 22, 562–8.

Closs, J. (1988) Patients sleep-wake rhythms in hospital. Parts 1 and 2,

Nursing Times 84, 1, 48–50 and 84, 2, 54–55.

Closs, S.J. and Cheater, F.M. (1994) Utilisation of nursing research: Culture, interest and support, *Journal of Advanced Nursing* 19, 762–73.

Cohen, L. and Mannion, L. (1985) *Research Methods in Education,* 2nd edn London, Routledge.

Crow, S., Rogers, J. and Larcombe, K. (1997) *Developing a Research Culture* London, English National Board.

Damle, A. (1989) Psychiatric aspects of sleep disorders in the elderly, *Geriatric Medicine* 19, 2, 67–73.

Department of Health (1991) *Research for Health: A research and development strategy for the NHS* London, HMSO.

Department of Health (1993) *Research for Health* London, HMSO.

Depoy, E. and Gitlin, L.N. (1994) *Introduction to Research Multiple Strategies for Health and Human Services* St Louis, Mosby.

Dias, B. (1992) Things that go bump, *Nursing Times* 88, 38, 36–8.

DiCenso, A. and Cullum, N (1998) Implementing evidence-based nursing: Some misconceptions, *Evidence-based Nursing* 1, 2, 38–40.

Dootson, S. (1990) Sensory imbalance and sleep loss. *Nursing Times* 86, 35, 26–9.

Dorociak, Y. (1990) Aspects of sleep, *Nursing Times* 86, 51, 38–40.

Dunwell, F. (1995) Insomnia and mental health, *Nursing Times* 91, 37, 31–2.

Duxbury, J. (1994a) Night nurses: Why are they undervalued? *Nursing Standard* 9, 11, 33–6.

Duxbury, J. (1994b) Avoiding disturbed sleep in hospitals. *Nursing Standard* 9, 10, 31–4.

Duxbury, J. (1994c) An investigation into primary nursing and its effect upon the nursing attitudes about the administration of prn night sedation, *Journal of Advanced Nursing* 19, 923–31.

Edell-Gustafsson, U., Aren, C., Hamrin, E. and Hetta, J. (1994) Nurses' notes on sleep patterns in patients undergoing coronary artery bypass surgery: A retrospective evaluation of nursing notes, *Journal of Advanced Nursing* 20, 331–6.

Ford, P. and Walsh, M. (1994) *New Rituals for Old: Nursing through the looking glass* Oxford, Butterworth-Heinemann Ltd.

Freak, L. (1995) Evaluating clinical trials, *Journal of Wound Care* 4, 3, 114–16.

George, B. (1985) Sleep and menopause, *Sleep Research* 14, 156.

Haddock, J. (1994) Reducing the effects of noise in hospital, *Nursing Standard* 8, 43, 25–8.

Halfens, R.J.G., Lendfers, M.L. and Cox, K. (1991) Sleep medication in Dutch Hospitals. *Journal of Advanced Nursing* 16, 1422–7.

Hayward, J. (1975) *Information: Prescription Against Pain* London, Royal College of Nursing.

Hill, J. (1989) A good night's sleep, *Senior Nurse* 9, 5, 17–19.

Hodgson, A. (1991) Why do we need sleep? Relating theory to practice, *Journal of Advanced Nursing* 16, 1503–10.

Hudson, R. (1994) Lavender oils aid relaxation in older patients (short report), *Nursing Times* 90, 30, 12.

Hunt, J. (1981) Indicators for nursing practice: The use of research findings, *Journal of Advanced Nursing* 6, 189–194.

Hunter, D.J. and Pollitt, C. (1992) Developments in health service research: Perspectives from Britain and the United States, *Journal of Public Health Medicine* 14, 2, 164–8.

Kearnes, S. (1989) Insomnia in the elderly, *Nursing Times* 85, 47, 32–3

Kemp, J. (1984) Nursing at night, *Journal of Advanced Nursing* 9, 2, 217–23.

King Edward's Hospital Fund for London (1960) *Noise Control in Hospitals*. London, King Edward's Fund.

Kitson, A. (1997) Using evidence to demonstrate the value of nursing, *Nursing Standard* 11, 28, 34–9.

Lloyd-Smith, W. (1996) Where's the evidence? *British Journal of Therapy and Rehabilitation* 3, 12, 659–61.

McClarey, M. (1997) Clinical effectiveness and evidence-based practice, *Nursing Standard* 11, 52, 33–7.

McCormack, M. and Whitehead, A. (1981) The effects of providing recreational activities on the engagement levels of long stay geriatric patients, *Age and Ageing* 10, 287–91.

McDonnell, A. (1998) Factors which may inhibit the utilisation of research findings in practice – and some solutions. In Crookes, P.A. and Davies, S. (eds) *Research into practice: Essential skills for reading and applying research in nursing and health care* Edinburgh, Balliere Tindall.

MacGregor, S.H. and Lannigan, N.A. (1992) The effect of the publication of guidelines on the prescription of benzodiazepines to acutely ill hospital in-patients, *Hospital Pharmacy Practice* 2, 8, 509–10.

MacGuire, J. (1990) Putting nursing research findings into practice: Research utilisation as an aspect of the management of change, *Journal of Advanced Nursing* 15, 614–20.

McMahon, A. (1996) Implications for nursing of the R&D funding policy, *Nursing Standard* 11, 28, 44–8.

Mantle, F. (1996) Sleepless and unsettled, *Nursing Times* 92, 23, 46–7

Marcus, N. (1995) Sleeping sickness, *Nursing Standard* 9, 22, 96.

Matthews, E.A., Farrell, G.A. and Blackmore, A.M. (1996) Effects of an environmental manipulation emphasising client centred care on agitation and sleep in dementia sufferers in a nursing home, *Journal of Advanced Nursing* 24, 439–47.

Muir Gray, J.A. (1997) *Evidenced-Based Healthcare: How to Make Heath Policy and Management Decisions* London, Churchill Livingstone.

NHS Centre for Reviews and Dissemination (1999) Getting evidence into practice, *Effective Health Care Bulletin* 5, 1 York, University of York.

Ogilvie, A. (1980) Sources and levels of noise on the ward at night, *Nursing Times* 76, 31, 1363–6.

Oswald, I. and Adam, K. (1983) *Get a Better Night's Sleep* London, Martin Dunitz.

Reagan, J. (1998) Will current clinical effectiveness initiatives encourage and facilitate practitioners to use evidence-based practice for the benefit of their clients? *Journal of Clinical Nursing* 7, 3, 244–50.

Rodgers, S. (1994) An exploratory study of research utilisation by nurses in general medical and surgical wards, *Journal of Advanced Nursing* 20, 904–11.

Shapiro, C.M. and Flanigan, M.J. (1993) Functions of sleep, *British Medical Journal* 306, 6874, 383–5.

Southwell, M. and Wistow, G. (1995a) Sleep in hospitals at night: Are patients' needs being met? *Journal of Advanced Nursing* 21, 1101–9.

Southwell, M. and Wistow, G. (1995b) In-patient sleep disturbance: The views of staff and patients, *Nursing Times* 91, 37, 29–31.

Stead, W. (1984) One awake, all awake! *Nursing Mirror* 160, 16, 20–1.

Tierney, A.J. (1987) Research issues: Putting research to good use, *Senior Nurse* 6, 3, 10.

Topf, M., Bookman, M. and Arand, D. (1996) Effects of critical care noise on the subjective quality of sleep, *Journal of Advanced Nursing* 24, 545–51.

Walsh, M. (1997) How nurses perceive barriers to research implementation, *Nursing Standard* 11, 29, 34–9.

Walsh, M. and Ford, P. (1989) *Nursing Rituals: Research and Rational Actions* Oxford, Heinemann Nursing.

Ward, C. (1992) From the other side, *Health Service Journal* 102, 5305, 26–7.

Webster, R.A. and Thompson, D.R. (1986) Sleep in hospital, *Journal of Advanced Nursing* 11, 447–57.

Wilkie, K. (1990) Golden slumbers . . . sleeplessness, *Nursing Times* 86, 51, 36–8.

Chapter 7

The importance of research dissemination and the barriers to implementation

Robert McSherry and Maxine Simmons

CONTENTS

Introduction

In this chapter ways of disseminating good practice, barriers to research implementation, and models for effective research appreciation and utilisation will be explored. The chapter provides an insight into the need for disseminating research findings and the barriers to achieving successful research utilisation. This will be reinforced by the use of reflective questions.

The importance of research dissemination

'Research that produces nothing but books will not suffice' (Lewins 1946). This emphasises the need to present research findings in a format that is assessable by all staff. The previous chapters describe the importance of generating evidence, being able to critically appraise the findings and to understand how evidence-based practice can enhance decision-making. The difficulty facing many nurses is acting on the evidence. How do we manage to put research findings into practice and/or share our findings with other colleagues?

Whilst the need for evidence-based nursing is now generally accepted, and evidence ultimately means research, nurses have little time to actually carry out research. For nursing to be informed by evidence – that is, informed by research findings – there is a need for relevant research. The research needs to be accessible to nurses who understand the need to inform their practice with research evidence and who have the critical appraisal skills to evaluate it, time to access it and skills to implement it.

There have, historically, been a number of barriers to nursing becoming a research-based profession (Hunt 1997). A fundamental problem is that nurses lack the skills and knowledge to read, interpret and understand research findings and there is a lack of recognition by managers of the need for nursing to be informed by evidence. Nursing research has often been seen as something undertaken by academic researchers and as much to do with the development of their academic career as with patient care. Traditionally, nursing has been seen as a practical occupation, with nurses providing care for patients under the general guidance of more senior nurses and the instructions of doctors. Nursing has been seen to require practical skills learnt from knowledgeable nurses and developed through experience. To the extent that nursing was based on scientific knowledge, this was 'borrowed' from other disciplines and taught to nurse as 'facts' to be accepted rather than knowledge to be evaluated before use. The skills and competencies taught were either based on nursing tradition (nursing knowledge accumulated experientially) or from medical research on what was clinically effective.

Training, then, prepared nurses to carry out practical tasks rather than to be knowledgeable reflective practitioners. This view of nursing was challenged, but it is only recently that nurse education has moved into Universities and nurses have been encouraged to learn the necessary skills and competencies to implement evidence-informed nursing. (This is not to suggest that much of the nursing knowledge that underpinned nursing practice was not based on sound research evidence, but that often the research findings that provided the evidence had been lost in the mists of time and nurses were unaware of them, or indeed of the need for nursing practice to be underpinned by a sound body of empirical research evidence.) Furthermore, nurse training did not equip nurses to access, assess or implement the findings of research.

However, even with the greater acceptance of the need for evidence-informed nursing, actually changing practice is complex and difficult. It is not easy to get those already engaged in nursing care to accept the need to reflect on the way that they provide care and seek the appropriate understanding of the evidence that underpins it and to change established practice where necessary.

The barriers to utilising nursing research are widespread and well documented in the literature (Hunt 1987, Bassett 1993, Cavanagh and Tross 1996, May *et al.* 1998), ranging from the nurse's lack of research awareness to organisational constraints (see Box 7.1).

Box 7.1 Barriers to research utilisation

- Lack of available research.
- Difficulties in accessibility.
- Lack of understanding.
- Attitudes towards research.
- Rituals and traditions v. problem solving approaches.
- Lack of confidence.
- Insufficient time.
- Educational issues.
- Organisational constraints.

In a 'Position Paper on Nursing Research' Greenwood offers two additional factors why research is not being used, factors which are easy to see but are always being overlooked.

Clinically nurses do not perceive research findings as relevant to their practice . . . they do not perceive them as relevant to their practice because frequently they are not relevant

(Greenwood 1984: 77)

Greenwood's paper may be accurate in stating that nurses' perceptions of research, and the relevance of the research may influence the individual nurse's ability to 'understand' and 'utilise' research findings in practice. Another major fundamental phenomenon seems to emerge: missing from Hunt's (1987) and Greenwood's (1984) literature is 'Pressure' from the government, UKCC and the media for nurses to use research findings to support clinical decision-making in order to improve the standards and quality of care offered to patients and carers. This situation has inadvertently increased the barriers to research utilisation because 'they are being pressurised from all angles to provide evidence-based practice without being given the skills and knowledge to do so. If nurses are not using research perhaps this is because they are basically unsure about what they know and feel about the whole issue' (McSherry 1997).

Perhaps one way of resolving some of the discussed barriers to research utilisation is by trying to answer the following questions.

Activity 7.1

The questions that needs answering are: What is the best way to disseminate or share good practice? What attributes are needed to support the sharing of good practice?

From experience as a Practice Development Adviser the following advice gives simple, but effective ways to enhance the sharing of good practices:

- Communication.
- Target audience.
- Presentation.
- Resources.
- Facilitation.

The above principles can be applied to disseminate the findings whether it is a research study or a literature review you have conducted.

Communication

Effective communication

Effective communication is essential if you are going to share your findings or areas of good practice with colleagues and must take into account some of the following points:

- Allow sufficient time for writing up and presenting the findings of your literature review.
- Seek expert senior nurse clarification in order to ensure the accuracy of the results/recommendations and to gain their support for the proposed change.
- When presenting the literature review findings, you need to consider any limitations to the review. Always be prepared for questions and discussions and for individuals to disagree with your conclusions/recommendations.
- Ensure that all staff are informed and involved with the review prior to, during and upon completion in order to maintain interest and have a feeling of shared ownership of the findings.
- When offering feedback, avoid the use of jargon and keep things simple in order for the audience to fully appreciate the advantages and disadvantages of your work.
- Communicate your intention to disseminate your research/review findings with all interested parties in order to ensure widespread dissemination and discussion associated with the results.
- Act upon feedback accordingly.

It is clear from the above points that communication is the essential attribute to ensuring effective dissemination of review findings.

Pediani and Walsh (2000) highlight the importance of effective communication through the use of simple repeatable messages.

Barriers to communication

Ineffective communication can easily lead to misinterpretations, misunderstandings and even a failure to utilise the findings in clinical practice from what might be a valuable contribution to nursing care. The barriers to ensuring effective communication include:

- Lack of time to effectively communicate with all individuals about the findings.
- Misinterpretation of recommendations due to complicated presentations. Some nurses may have limited understanding of research and may not understand or may feel threatened by research jargon (keep things simple).
- Inability to access information. This point links with the target audience and the need to share the information from the review using methods that are appropriate to the individuals you wish to inform.

Target audience

Integral to research dissemination is the notion that the individuals who have reviewed or are intending to review practices consider how, when and to whom the feedback of the findings will be given. The term 'target audience' comes to mind. It is essential to consider who you are going to feedback your findings to. Are you aiming to share your review findings within the nursing team, directorate or to the organisation where you work? Are the staff junior, senior or management? The answer to these questions should influence the nature of your feedback.

If presenting to the nursing team, it may be sufficient to take a 20-minute slot at a team meeting to feedback or, alternatively, provide the staff with a summary fact sheet of the key points gained from the course or research. To the senior staff or directorate you might distribute an information sheet along with a report of the review findings and how this may enhance patient care. For senior managers or commissioning authority you would want to provide an in-depth report, along with an oral presentation and recommendations for change and cost involvement if necessary.

If you would like to share your ideas with the wider nursing audience, it may be possible to provide a summary/report for the Royal College of Nursing (RCN), English National Board (ENB) or United Kingdom Central Council for Nursing, Midwifery and Health Visiting (UKCC) research or interest groups that is specific to your subject area or relevant to your findings.

It is important to make contact with the relevant parties before sending any information. An important point to remember is to keep a record of to whom, when and how you shared your findings so that monitoring of progress of dissemination to the target group(s) can be undertaken.

Presentation

If you have taken the time and energy to communicate your proposed ideas for change and designed and implemented a good research review, don't fall at the last hurdle!

Make sure that you write up and present your results in a clear, concise and logical manner (Effective Communication). The 'research process' is defined as 'a framework made up of a sequence of logical steps within which research is carried out. It provides a chronological list of the tasks to be done in order to successfully complete a research project. This framework can be used as headings in writing up your research review' (Parahoo and Reid 1988). (See Appendix, p. 149.) It is essential to establish what is the best way to present and disseminate your findings, paying attention to the style and type of presentation, for example, oral or written is essential. A combination of oral presentation (team meeting/ conference) and written presentation (poster/paper) may be the most effective. Points to bear in mind are as follows:

- What is the best way to get over your results most effectively? Poster, oral presentation or written report, or combination of all?
- Think about the audience you want to inform, about whether it is the public or other colleagues because the style and nature of presentation may be significantly different.

- If you are considering publishing your results in a journal, contact that specific journal and ask for their guide to publishing information sheet in order to assist you in this process.
- Utilise computer software packages that are available to aid with visual presentation and designs.
- Ensure if using audio visual aids that you are competent and prepared to deal with unexpected technical failures.

Please remember that having successfully undertaken an effective literature review, systematic review or a meta analysis of the literature, the last thing you want to do is to contribute to the barriers against research utilisation by not sharing and disseminating your findings, making the findings inaccessible to colleagues, over-use of jargon, etc. If you are apprehensive or lack confidence or experience (we all have that concern at the start) to share your findings, there is always someone out there to support you. For example:

- clinical audit/research department;
- practice and professional development advisers;
- research and development advisers;
- university lecturers/researchers;
- your peers and line managers.

Resources

This is a big issue that affects the sharing and dissemination of new innovations. It costs money in terms of release time:

- for staff to undertake and present finding of their reviews;
- for the target audience to attend feedback or become involved with any innovations;
- to present at a local or national conference;
- to design and present a poster.

To prepare for a conference or poster presentation will require financial support for such things as audio visual aids, travel, etc.

It is difficult to find time for writing for publication, especially if you are trying to do a job at the same time, or have social commitments, etc. Additionally, you may have to consider the cost implications for changing practices following a research study or review of practice. In order to avoid disappointment after completing a review that you want to share with colleagues, it is essential to consider prior to the review the potential financial implications and sources of funding:

- Consult with your managers to see if they are prepared to support the costs associated with your proposed practice change. Managers have a responsibility to ensure that services demonstrate value for money. Therefore if your proposed change(s) in practice could improve efficiency and effectiveness of the service, you are more likely to be successful in securing financial support and realising the time to pursue your review and subsequent dissemination.
- Consult with other departments to see if any facilities exist within the organisation to aid you. For example, medical illustrations or medical photography department, clinical audit departments, etc.
- Utilise the expertise within your local clinical area.
- Negotiate access to computer facilities and word processing.
- Collaborate with the local university school of health, research units to offer academic support, etc.
- Negotiate time out from your post in order to ensure that you have the time, motivation, commitment and support to do the review effectively to reduce the pressures of insufficient time.

In summary, it is essential that the barriers to research utilisation are resolved in order to ensure that the findings are used in practice. For reviews to be undertaken and not be communicated to a wider audience could be seen to be contributing to the theory–practice gap. The failure of nurses to implement into practice their review findings is in itself a barrier to research utilisation. Having explored the barriers to research utilisation and ways of dissemination, it is imperative to briefly introduce the concept of change management which is associated with any changes in practice.

Facilitation

The final aspect of ensuring successful implementation of evidence-informed practice is facilitation. Facilitation 'is a technique by which one person makes things easier for others' (Heron 1989). The difference between a facilitator and an opinion leader is that facilitators 'consciously use a series of interpersonal and group skills to achieve change whereas opinion leaders may influence more because of their status and technical competence' (Kitson *et al.* 1998). Kitson *et al.* identify the necessity of facilitation in achieving and maintaining evidence-informed development in practice. It is important to be aware that you may not have the time or skills to facilitate the implementation of change and should seek the advice and guidance of a recognised facilitator in your organisation, or external bodies if required.

Change management models

When changing practice based on the findings of research, the nurse may need to manage resistance which, without an awareness of change management strategies, may create difficulties in successfully implementing the research findings. This section briefly explores frameworks for implementing change, strategies for managing resistance and an understanding of the role of the change agent.

The statement below by Machiavelli reflects the difficulties faced by nurses embarking upon making changes in practice:

There is nothing more difficult to carry out, nor more doubtful of success, nor more dangerous to handle than a new order of things. For the reformer has enemies in all those who profit by the old order, and only lukewarm defenders in all those who would profit by the new order, this lukewarmness arising partly from fear of their adversaries who have the laws in their favour, and partly from the incredulity of mankind, who do not truly believe in anything new until they have actual experience of it.

The above highlights the difficulties associated with changing practices and in changing individual and organisational behaviours.

The first step in implementing a successful change is to correctly identify what the problem is as discussed in Chapter 5. The nurse needs to answer one or more of the following questions:

- What is the problem that requires a change to be made? (Anderson 1991)
- 'What changes are needed in my place of work to make it function more effectively?' (Anderson 1991)
- What are the implications for changing my practice based on the available evidence?

To enable the nurse to make an accurate diagnosis of the situation, the work area requires systematic examination. A useful tool to perform this examination is the Nadler and Tushman diagnostic model (Anderson 1991). See Figure 7.1.

Examination of the situation in this systematic manner enables the nurse to identify where the problem stems from. As each of the components effects each other, it is also possible to identify other factors that may be contributing to the problem and require incorporating into the planned change. For more information on this subject read: Anderson, E. (1991) *Book 9. Managing Change. Managing Health Services* Oxford: The Open University.

Having identified the area of practice requiring change where do you go from here. There are many change models available to aid this process; below is one example.

A change model

Change is a complex process inherent with barriers which threaten the successful implementation of the research findings. Utilising a change model can help guide the change process and help to reduce obstacles which may be encountered. Lewins (cited in Allen 1993) proposes a change model, which has three fundamental stages :

- Unfreezing.
- Moving.
- Refreezing.

Unfreezing

For change to occur individuals need to recognise that there is a need for change. Lewins' force-field theory suggests that for unfreezing to occur there is a need to understand that driving and

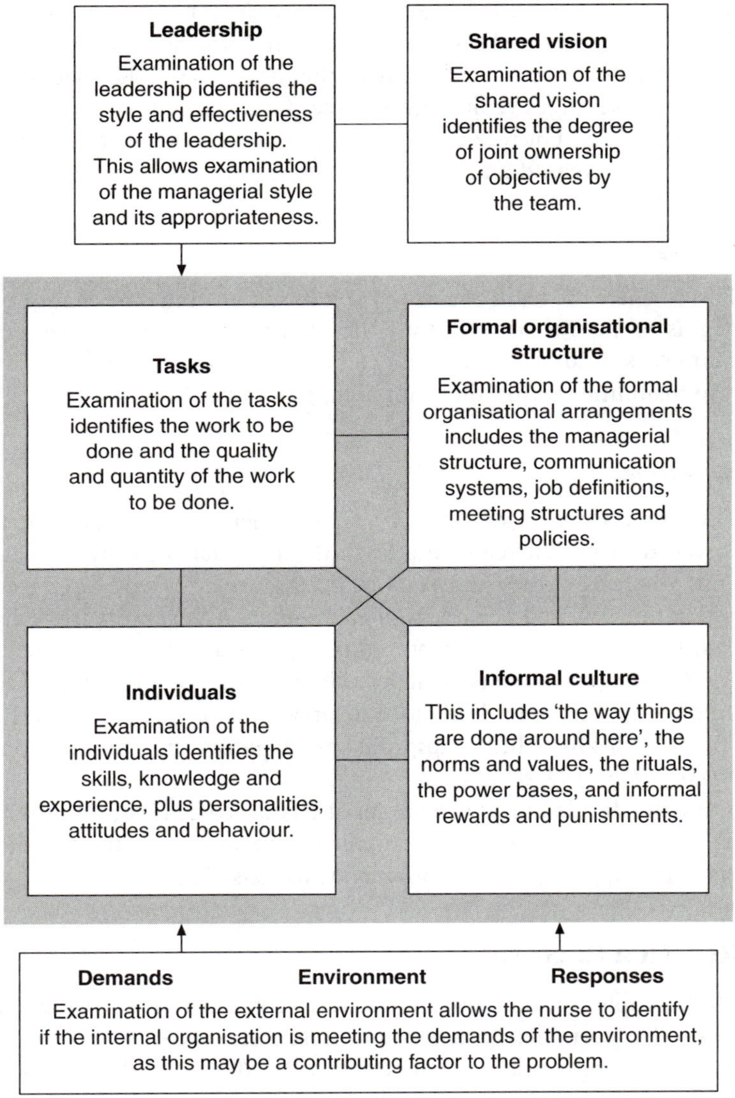

Leadership	Shared vision
Examination of the leadership identifies the style and effectiveness of the leadership. This allows examination of the managerial style and its appropriateness.	Examination of the shared vision identifies the degree of joint ownership of objectives by the team.

Tasks	Formal organisational structure
Examination of the tasks identifies the work to be done and the quality and quantity of the work to be done.	Examination of the formal organisational arrangements includes the managerial structure, communication systems, job definitions, meeting structures and policies.

Individuals	Informal culture
Examination of the individuals identifies the skills, knowledge and experience, plus personalities, attitudes and behaviour.	This includes 'the way things are done around here', the norms and values, the rituals, the power bases, and informal rewards and punishments.

Demands   Environment   Responses

Examination of the external environment allows the nurse to identify if the internal organisation is meeting the demands of the environment, as this may be a contributing factor to the problem.

Figure 7.1   Nadler and Tushman's diagnostic model.

Source: Nadler, D. and Tushman, M.L. (1977) *Perspectives on Behaviour* New York, McGraw Hill. Reprinted from *Evidence-Based Healthcare*, Nadler, D. and Tushman, M.L., table 4.1, p. 61 (1997), by permission of the publisher Churchill Livingstone.

restraining forces exist. For example, a driving force may be the evidence to support a change in practice and the restraining forces could be negative attitudes from the staff about the evidence. Whilst these forces remain in balance the situation will remain in the *status quo*. Unfreezing of a situation can occur when driving forces are increased and restraining forces decreased.

Moving

This is where the team begins to explore and examine the change or begins to accept or adjust to the changes being implemented. Teamwork needs to be nurtured and the emergence of key roles and responsibilities within the team highlighted.

Refreezing

This often occurs after a period of time when the change has been accepted within the team and the staff settle back into a functional unit, where key roles and responsibilities are adopted, supported and communicated to and from each other. An example from my own personal experience where this happened was when the staff and I developed patients' relatives' clinics which required changes in practice to be made. For more information read: McSherry, R. (1996) Multidisciplinary approaches to patient communication, *Nursing Times* 92, 8, 42–3.

Having decided upon the model of change to be used, it is essential to be aware of how individuals may react or respond to your plans to implement a particular evidence-based practice.

Reaction to change

Most people find change disruptive and by merely exposing the flaws of a particular practice and presenting research findings to support the rationale for change you will still most likely face resistance. Although a change may have the same indications for individuals to resist, people will respond differently. There are four main reasons why people resist change (Kotter and Schlesinger 1979):

- *Parochial Self Interest* – Where individuals may resist because they fear they may lose something they value as a result of the change.
- *Misunderstanding and Lack of Trust* – Individuals often resist change because they do not understand its implications and perceive it might cost them more than they have to gain. This may occur where there is trust lacking between the person initiating the change and the workforce.
- *Different Assessments* – Individuals may assess the situation differently from those initiating the change and see more costs than benefits as a result, not only for themselves but for the organisation as a whole.
- *Low Tolerance for Change* – Individuals may fear they will not be able to develop the new skills or behaviour needed after the change.

The potential varied responses by individuals to a change in practice may be anticipated by analysing individual personality types in relation to their reaction to change. Allen (1993) provides an illustration of Lancaster and Lancaster's (1982) adaptation of Rogers and Shoemaker personality type categories (Table 7.1) which can aid the nurse in predicting the probable response of individuals to a suggested change.

Table 7.1 Personality types identified by Rogers and Shoemaker

Personality type	Personality traits
Innovators	Curious, enthusiastic and eager.
Early adapters	Moderately enthusiastic, well-established group members, high self-esteem. Do not usually introduce radical/controversial ideas.
Early majority	Accept the innovation just before the majority do.
Late majority	View the innovation with scepticism, do not actively resist.
Laggards	Suspicious of change, discourage others by their negative attitude.
Rejecters	Openly reject change and encourage others to do so.

Source: Adapted from Lancaster, J. and Lancaster, W. (1982) *The Nurse as the Change Agent* St Louis, Mosby

Let us explore our own personality in relation to potential change by working on Activity 7.2

Activity 7.2 Reflective exercise

● What is your personality type?
● Do you react differently depending on the change being implemented?
● Think of some changes you have opposed. Why did you oppose them?
● Are there changes you have actively supported? Why were you in favour of them?

If you are considering changing practice based around evidence, it is essential to perform the above personality analysis in order to establish where the resistance to change may exist and which individuals may be supportive of the change. It is particularly important to identify those individuals who have the ability to influence other members of the team or resource allocation.

Key individuals

Key individuals are people whose co-operation, or lack of resistance is essential if the planned implementation of the research findings is to be successful. Key individuals are those who have the information needed to design the change and those individuals whose co-operation is essential to enable the change to move forward. Through identifying key individuals and their level of commitment to the change, the nurse is able to plan appropriate strategies to increase or decrease their commitment appropriately. Through analysing the current situation (see Nadler and Tushman's diagnostic model, Figure 7.1), it is possible to identify who the key individuals are who need to be involved in the change and also those (internal and external) who are effected by the change. The position of the nurse in relation to key individuals is important when attempting to influence their behaviour. The power base of the relationship will determine which change strategy the nurse should choose and whose co-operation they need to secure to help influence others.

Handy hint

Do not under estimate the effect of implementing research findings. Making a change can be compared to throwing a pebble into a still pond – it may only be small but the ripples it makes spread across the pond.

An innovator may be described as being an individual who generates ideas, introduces innovation, develops a climate for change by overcoming resistance and understanding forces for acceptance, and implements and evaluates change (Vaughan and Pilmore 1992). Without the presence of the innovator and their support of the change process, the innovation will not take place as all these attributes are essential for the implementation of successful innovation.

Innovators do not need to be the most senior people, but they do require the power to implement change (Allen 1993). The position of the innovator in relation to key individuals is important when attempting to change individuals' behaviour. The relationship of the innovator to key individuals will determine which change strategy the innovator should choose. Where the innovator has little or no influence with key individuals, they need to seek the support of colleagues who are able to influence others where necessary.

For example

The nurse needs to identify their power bases in relation to key individuals. The power base held by the innovator will determine which change strategies they can successfully utilise. French and Raven (1959) identify five sources of power, see Table 7.2 below:

Table 7.2 Five sources of power

Power	Type
Physical power	The power of superior force.
Resource power	Control of resources which are desired by others.
Position power	The power attached to a role or status.
Expert power	The power vested in an individual because of their acknowledged expertise. (Can only be given by others and may be situation dependent.)
Personal power	Linked to charisma and popularity.

Kotter and Schlesinger (1979) identify six different strategies that can be utilised to influence a change in behaviour (Table 7.3). When planning the change, the nurse may need to utilise a variety of strategies dependent upon the situation, reason for resistance and power bases available. When planning to implement the research findings, the nurse needs to determine the type of resistance anticipated and try to understand the reasons why. The nurse needs to determine if key individuals will be supportive and co-operative, that is, innovators, early adapters. If it is anticipated that key individuals will not be supportive, strategies for influencing their behaviour need to be implemented prior to commencing the change.

Activity 7.3 Reflective exercise

- Consider a change you have initiated or been affected by.
- What types of resistance did staff demonstrate towards the change?
- What do you think were the reasons for staff resistance to the change?
- What change strategies do you think were used?
- Which types of power bases did the change agent possess and use?
- Were the change strategies employed successful in ensuring implementation of the change?
- Give your reasons why the strategies used may have been successful or unsuccessful.

Table 7.3 Change strategies

Change strategy	Power base	Rationale	Situation
Education and communication	Expert and personal power	Communicating ideas helps people to understand the reason for the change.	Useful where resistance is based on misunderstanding. Requires that the resisters have trust in the innovator.
Participation and involvement	Personal power	Through being involved in designing the change, the change participants develop ownership of the change and become committed to its implementation.	Useful where the resisters have the information needed to design the change and also have a lot of power to resist the change.
Facilitation and support	Expert and personal power	Providing training, understanding how individuals feel and providing emotional support can help to reduce individuals' fears related to the change.	Useful where individuals' resistance is due to fear of adapting to new roles.
Negotiation and agreement	Resource power	Resistance may be reduced by offering incentives.	Useful where an individual/group is going to lose out as a result of the change and also has the power to resist the implementation.
Manipulation and co-option	Resource power	Involves giving an individual/group a perception of increased status or reward in return for their co-operation.	Useful where there is inadequate time/resources to implement more costly strategies.
Explicit and implicit coercion	Position power	Involves the innovator forcing the resistors to adhere to the change. May result in long-term resentment towards the innovation which may effect the long-term success of the change.	Useful where speed is essential.

Source: Adapted from Kotter, J.P. and Schlesinger, L.A. (1979)

A major factor in ensuring successful innovation is managing resistance, which involves dealing with people and their feelings. To carry out this role innovators need to be socially aware and possess good interpersonal skills. The innovator also requires stamina, as the change process can be frustrating, requiring persistence and flexibility to overcome problems (Allen 1993). The role of the innovator is one of the major factors influencing the effectiveness of a change and both the innovator and participants need to understand the role to minimise conflict and tension (Vaughan and Pilmore 1992). The innovator may come from within or outside of the workplace where the change is required. Advantages and disadvantages of both internal and external innovators are illustrated in Table 7.4.

Table 7.4 Internal and external innovators

	Advantages	Disadvantages
Internal innovator	In-depth understanding of the situation. Knowledge of the systems and understanding of the workforce.	May be biased when making judgements due to having a vested interest in the situation. Workforce may be effected by previous change failures of the innovator.
External innovator	More open-minded. Little personally to gain through the change. More able to see the situation clearly. Less likely to be biased.	Does not have a deep understanding of the situation. Will need to gain the trust and confidence of the workforce.

Source: Vaughan, B. and Pilmore, M. 1992, Allen 1993.

Activity 7.4 Reflective excercise is designed to enable you to identify good and/or poor practices related to evidence-based practice changes.

Activity 7.4 Reflective exercise

- Consider a change you have been involved in either as a change agent or where your practice has been effected by a change.
- Was the change based on any evidence?
- Was the change agent internal or external?
- Was the change agent the appropriate person to implement the change?
- Give reasons for your answer to the above question.

Conclusion

In order to be able to appreciate the possible benefits of research in aiding us to practise evidence-informed nursing, it is essential that we familiarise ourselves with the best ways to share our findings, along with the barriers that may prevent individuals or organisations from adapting to change. From our experience, changes which have the potential to improve care and where there is strong evidence for the change in practice can often still be viewed negatively, for example, by the named qualified nurse, team or primary nursing staff.

In order to respond positively rather than negatively to evidence-based change, it is essential for us to establish our own personality type or possible response to change, key areas covered within this chapter. Remember, 'not all change is improvement but all improvement is change' (Berwick 1996).

Summary of key points

- To ensure evidence informs practice it is important to effectively communicate your review findings.
- To practise evidence-informed nursing the barriers to using research to support evidence need to be managed.
- Successful, maintained change in practice is achieved through rigorous planning and thoughtful facilitation.

Recommended reading

Allen, A. (1993) Changing theory in nursing practice, *Senior Nurse* 13, 1, Jan/Feb, 43–6

Kitson, A., Harvey, G. and McCormack, B. (1998) Enabling the implementation of evidence-based practice; A conceptual framework, *Quality in Healthcare* 7, 149–58.

The Foundation of Nursing Studies (1996) *Reflection for Action,* London, The Foundation of Nursing Studies.

Pediani, R. and Walsh, M. (2000) Changing practice: Are memes the answer? *Nursing Standard* 14, 24, 36–40.

References

Allen, A. (1993) Changing theory in nursing practice, *Senior Nurse* 13, 1, Jan/Feb, 43–46.

Anderson, E. (1991) *Book 9 Managing Health Services* Milton Keynes, The Open University.

Bassett, C. (1993) Nurse teachers' attitudes to research: A phenomenological study, *Journal of Advanced Nursing* 19, 1–8.

Berwick, D. (1996) A primer in leading the improvement of systems, *BMJ* 312, 619–22.

Bor, R. and Watts, M. (1993) Talking to patients about sexual matters, *British Journal of Nursing* 2, 13, 657–61.

Cavanagh, J.S. and Tross, G. (1996) Utilizing research findings in nursing: Policy and practice considerations, *Journal of Advanced Nursing* 24, 1077–82.

Crookes, P.A. (1992) Professional care in health. In Buddy, J. and Rice, V. (eds) *Perspectives and Practices* Palmerston North, Dunmore Press.

Foundation of Nursing Studies (1996) *Reflection for Action,* London, The Foundation of Nursing Studies.

French, J. and Raven, B. (1959) The basis of social power. In Cartwright D. (ed.) *Studies in Social Power* Annarbor, University of Michigan, Institute for Social Research.

Greenwood, J. (1984) Nursing research: A position paper, *Journal of Advanced Nursing* 6, 189–94.

Heron, J. (1989) *The Facilitators Handbook* London, Kogan Page.

Hunt, J. (1981) Indicators for nursing practice: The use of research findings, *Journal of Advanced Nursing* 6, 189–94.

Hunt, J. (1997) Towards evidence based practice, *Nursing Management* 4, 2, 14–17.

Hunt, M. (1987) The process of translating research findings into practice, *Journal of Advanced Nursing* 12, 101–10.

Kitson, A., Harvey, G. and McCormack, B. (1998) Enabling the implementation of evidence based practice: A conceptual framework, *Quality in Healthcare* 7, 149–58.

Kotter, J.P. and Schlesinger, L.A. (1979) Choosing strategies for change, *Harvard Business Review* 57, 2, Mar/Apr, 106–15.

Lewins, K. (1946) Action research and minority problems, *Journal of Social Issues* 2, 34–6.

May, A., Alexander, C. and Mulhall, A. (1998) Research utilisation in nursing: Barriers and opportunities, *Journal Clinical Effectiveness* 3, 2, 59–63.

McSherry, R. (1996) Multidisciplinary approaches to patient communication, *Nursing Times* 92, 8, 42–3.

McSherry, R. (1997) What do registered nurses and midwives feel and know about research? *Journal of Advanced Nursing* 25, 985–98.

Nadler, D. and Tushman, M.L. (1977) *Perspectives of Behaviour* New York, McGraw-Hill.

Parahoo, K. and Reid, W. (1988) Research skills 5: Critical reading of research, *Nursing Times* 84, 69–72.

Pediani, R. and Walsh, M. (2000) Changing practice: Are memes the answer? *Nursing Standard* 14, 24, 36–40.

Vaughan, B. and Pilmore, M. (1992) *Managing Nursing Work* London, Scutari Press.

Weston, A. (1993) Challenging assumptions, *Nursing Times* 89, 18, 26–9.

Chapter 8
Conclusion
The way forward

Robert McSherry and Maxine Simmons

This book has introduced the term evidence-informed nursing in order to distinguish the relationship between evidence and practice in nursing from that in medicine, where evidence has come to be mainly associated with high quality randomised control trials (RCT). We argue that there can be high quality evidence from research other than that based on RCT and that the nurse must evaluate all evidence for relevance and appropriateness.

At this point we hope you will have an understanding of what we mean by evidence-informed nursing and will have developed some of the skills necessary to enable you to utilise high quality research findings in your professional practice. Development of the core skills of research awareness, critical appraisal, reflection, and implementation and evaluation of change are fundamental skills which are relevant to all aspects of nursing ranging from clinical practice, management and education through to professional development. By using the framework of evidence-informed practice suggested in this book and by applying the skills in practice, you will enable not only yourself but nursing as a profession to be recognised as modern and fit for its practice and purpose. The following examples show some of the areas in which evidence-informed nursing could benefit the wider nursing agenda and help realise the government's aim of modernising health care.

Professionalisation

Nursing historically has struggled to develop recognition as a profession at least in part because of the lack of a discrete knowledge base. In the practice setting, the recognition of nurses by other health care professionals as fellow professionals has been hindered by the lack of a unique body of knowledge to underpin practice. Furthermore, where nursing knowledge has been developed and implemented in practice it has often not withstood critical review by other professions on the grounds of a lack of scientific rigour. Evidence-informed nursing addresses both these issues. The processes it requires not only facilitate a research mindedness equal to that of scientifically based professions such as medicine, but also includes core critical skills, such as reflection, that have not traditionally been part of medical training. Evidence-informed nursing provides nurses with the confidence to know that the evidence-based changes in practice they have introduced will withstand critical review by their peers and other professional colleagues.

Autonomy

In the past medicine was seen to treat and nurses to care. Nurses were not seen and did not see themselves as autonomous practitioners. The development of nursing research and knowledge now enables nurses not only to deliver care, but also to prescribe nursing treatment/interventions independently of medicine, for example wound care. This trend will continue as nurses use the processes identified within the evidence-informed cycle to further enhance the care they deliver. As more independent therapeutic nursing interventions are introduced following rigorous scientific review, nurses' autonomy will also increase. This is particularly important as we witness the introduction of new roles such as that of Nurse Consultant. The Department of Health documents (DOH 1997, 2000) lay out the government's intention for modernisation of health care. Within these strategies nursing has a major role to play in developing new, smarter ways of delivering care. Evidence-informed nursing and its association with practicing evidence-based nursing can enable nurses to grasp these opportunities, further developing their autonomy and clinical expertise.

Nursing theory and practice

The evidence-informed cycle offers nursing a framework that facilitates the integration of theory into practice for individuals, teams or organisations. Its use over time should assist in narrowing the perceived gap between theory and practice (McSherry 2000). For evidence-based nursing to become a reality, cultural and attitudinal changes are required in the way research is viewed to support practice. Evidence-informed nursing attempts to address these issues by providing the core skills necessary to enable nurses to view research more positively and to understand how it contributes to practice. In our experience clinical staff are well aware of the need to use research to support practice and know that using research can make positive changes in clinical care. However, this can only be achieved by equipping people with the knowledge, skills and competence to critically appraise research and by developing the supporting processes necessary to enable successful practice in current or new roles. At the same time, employers need to encourage staff to express their views, highlighting difficulties or concerns over their practices or in meeting new challenges. Such approaches can only be fostered by robust systems of communication where honesty and openness are at the heart of discussion.

This text will ensure that you are informed of the core skills and have the knowledge to enable you to meet the challenges of practising evidence-informed nursing in the future, as new knowledge is developed and old knowledge is challenged. Evidence-informed nursing supports the government's clinical governance agenda by encouraging staff to develop or provide practices based upon the most appropriate evidence. To practise within the clinical governance frameworks, the ability to critique research and learn from the challenges of everyday practices – whether good or not so good – is a key component of the government's health care modernisation agenda. The application of the skills and learning gained from the content of this text can only serve you well for the future and will help you to deliver quality care to patients and their carers.

Good Luck

Robert McSherry, Maxine Simmons and Pamela Abbott

The Editors

References

Department of Health (1997) *Modern Dependable* London, Stationery Office.
Department of Health (2000) *The National Plan* London, Stationery Office.
McSherry, R. (2000) Is there a great divide between nursing theory and practice? *Nursing Times* 96, 17, 16.

Appendix

An example of critical appraisal undertaken using a framework similar to those described by Andrew F. Long, carried out by Carol Suter during her undergraduate studies 1998.

Research Article: McSherry, R. (1997) What do registered nurses and midwives feel and know about research, *Journal of Advanced Nursing* 25, 985–98.

Research assignment
Critique of a research paper

Outlined in the recent government white paper *The New NHS Modern, Dependable* (Department of Health (DoH) 1997), special attention was paid to nurses providing evidence-based practice for patients. Prior to this, *The Strategy for Research in Nursing, Midwifery and Health Visiting* (DoH 1993) placed a responsibility on nurses to become research literate. As nurses continue their battle to gain recognition as a professional body, utilisation and recognition of research seems to provide one of the ways forward (Dyson 1996). Despite this, few nurses are involved in research and their knowledge remains poor (Leighton-Beck 1997). The piece of research I aim to critique questions what registered nurses and midwives feel and know about research.

After scrutinising several frameworks for critiquing a research study (Hawthorne 1983, Clarke 1994 and Hek 1996), I have decided in this assignment to use the guidelines outlined by Burns and Grove (1997) and Cormack (1996). I will, however, borrow some characteristics from some of the other frameworks.

The title of the research article which I have chosen to critique is as follows:

'What do registered nurses and midwives feel and know about research?'

The research paper was published in the *Journal of Advanced Nursing* in 1997 and the research was performed by Mr R. McSherry, a Nursing Lecturer and Practice Development Adviser in Chesterfield, Derbyshire. From reading the title of the research and the details of the author, one can speedily deduce the characteristics and requirements of them both (Cormack 1996, Burns and Grove 1997). It gives a clear impression of what the study is about and also confirms that the author of the study is well placed and qualified to carry out the research in question.

Mr McSherry is a registered general nurse and all his qualifications are nursing related. This piece of research was performed towards his Masters degree, and at present he is studying towards a PhD and is conducting research in a similar field, looking at evidence-based practice and, in particular, nurse attitudes. Mr McSherry was contacted with a view to examining the questionnaire used in the research. He offered his help with any other queries and the above information has been obtained by telephoning Mr R. McSherry.

Abstract

An abstract summarises the contents of a piece of work and gives the reader the opportunity to decide if the article/paper is relevant to their particular needs or of interest to them. It should include all essentials that allow readers to grasp what a study is about (Polit and Hungler 1991). The abstract comprehensively and concisely covers all that it should. It identifies the research problem, outlines the methodology and gives details of the sample subjects. It then goes on to report the major findings of the study (Polit and Hungler 1991, Burns and Grove 1997, Cormack 1996).

Introduction

The study is introduced under the heading 'The Study Background' and discussed in this section are the legitimate professional documents which indicate that research has an important part to play in nurses' professionalism, their commitment to patients and their accountability to the United Kingdom Central Council for Nurses (UKCC) (*Working for Patients* DoH 1989, *The Patients Charter: Raising the Standard* DoH 1992, UKCC 1992). The introduction acquaints readers with the research problem and also with the context within which it was formulated (Polit and Hunger 1991) and as Mr R. McSherry has 'set the scene', the rationale for the study clearly enfolds (Cormack 1996).

Literature review

The literature review is comprehensive and up-to-date and also includes fundamental work from as early as 1946. It presents a balanced view of the literature and clearly portrayed are the arguments supporting the need for a wider knowledge-base for nurses with regards to research. In contrast, the written views regarding why nurses still do not use research effectively and the reasons behind this lack of utility are also highlighted.

It is acknowledged that few studies have been carried out in relation to what nurses 'know and feel' about research and the two studies that are included in the literature review are discussed and analysed. Funk *et al.*'s study (1991, cited in McSherry 1997) looked at why barriers occurred in the use of research and Stokes (1981, cited in McSherry 1997) produced a study where 64 per cent of staff nurses who were sampled from 23 hospitals in the United States believed that finding results from nursing research was not reflected in their patient care.

The hypothesis

The research does not have a hypothesis, it has a research question which is clearly identified in the title.

Methodology

Questionnaires were chosen as the method of collecting data. The entire nursing work-force within the study's hospital were chosen to take part in the study, a total of 765 nurses and midwives. In quantitative research sampling procedures are less rigidly prescribed as in qualitative data (Coyne 1997). The author of this research believes that it could be argued that this sample is a cluster sample of the total UK population of nurses. The questionnaires adopted an additional survey design and thus ensured that the questions were ordered to obtain the most important information first.

Questionnaires as a method of collecting data enable the researcher to reach numerous people very quickly, either through self-administration or by post. They can be analysed easily (depending on the design) and in cases of a sensitive nature, or in this instance embarrassment due to lack of knowledge, honest answers can be given. An important point is that the larger the sample for the research study, the more likely it is that the researcher will be able to generalise (however, in this case generalisation of the results is limited and acknowledged) (Clifford and Cough 1990).

A well-designed questionnaire allows the respondent to progress from one question to the next with ease in a sequence which appears logical. This sequence may differ greatly from the order which is most pleasing to the researcher (Cormack 1996). The questionnaire under scrutiny appears logically laid out and can be completed with ease. Cormack (1996) refers to funnelling questions, asking the most general questions first as a preamble to successively more specific questions. This questionnaire was designed to obtain the important information first and has succeeded by obtaining that information. This fact may be because the questions asked were not of a conflicting nature.

Questionnaires have been referred to as an interrogation protocol by Ackerman and Lyons (1981), probably due to the fact that they give no opportunity for conversation and are totally devised to obtain maximum information. This questionnaire, however, incorporated fixed-response questions with open spaces for comments to support the results with written, factual qualitative evidence.

Pilot study

A pilot study is advocated to analyse the research method chosen and can be used to develop a research plan. It gives the opportunity to try out data analysis techniques, to refine tools of research, to determine whether or not the proposed study is feasible and identify any problems with the design. It is also used to examine the reliability and validity of the research instrument (Ogier 1992).

In order to enhance the validity and reliability of this research a pilot study was undertaken in which 25 questionnaires were completed by out-patients staff and practice development advisers. Their comments were invited as regards to the suitability of the questionnaires, and as a result minor changes were made. There are advantages to using questionnaires as previously discussed, but devising a questionnaire that is both valid and reliable takes time and skill (Hek 1995).

The results of the pilot study were comparable with the main study but the obvious difference was in the response rate, which was 84 per cent in the pilot study and only 36.33 per cent in the main study. The participants in the pilot study were approached personally and they had three weeks to complete the questionnaire. The participants of the main study only had two weeks to complete the questionnaire and, because of the enormity of the sample size, invitation into the study was done via letter. Also incorporated into the main study were part-time workers. These differences and limitations are acknowledged in the paper.

Results and data presentation

Prior to presenting the findings of the study, the author of the work has explained which method of data collection was used. When contacted by telephone, Mr McSherry informed me that a statistician was not employed to assist him, but that he has a sound statistical base knowledge and the analysis of the data was undertaken with the aid of SPSS Word for Windows. With regards to attitudes and understanding, a 'Measurement Rating Scale' was designed. Chi-squared (χ^2) and correlation (cross-tabulation) tests were applied to the data to see if any association existed between the variables. The findings from these are hard to follow, not due to their presentation but only due to the inexperience of the author, who has to refer to relevant literature to assist. What the findings reveal is that the correlation between two quantitative variables are not chance findings, and that the findings are of significance (Hicks 1990).

The main study results have been put across to the reader in several different ways. Pie charts have been chosen by the author to portray, for example, how many questionnaires were distributed to each directorate and also the response in terms of grade and length of qualification. The charts were then supported by descriptive data. Response by directorate is displayed in a table format which is particularly easy to follow, and in most of the data presentation both raw figures and percentages are stated, which seems to have more impact. The arithmetic of the results is correct in every way. Numbers tally and percentages are not rounded off, they are given to a decimal point and when checked appear to be completely correct.

There is much descriptive data which can be absorbed with little effort. It is also logically presented which assists the reader even further. A graph is used to present the details of where research training was received and, again, this has been supported by descriptive data. The use of the variety of methods of data presentation have assisted in making the reading of study results more interesting and using more than one method for certain data has improved the understanding.

Discussion

The poor response rate obviously caused some disappointment and it is supported by literature which gives one possible explanation for it. It gives a further breakdown of the sample details which aims to give the rationale behind some of the findings. These balanced descriptions of the main findings are constantly supported by relevant literature. One of the points that became evident throughout the research was that research-based practice cannot be achieved without the support, supervision and co-operation of managers and peers. These prerequisites to nursing research are pointed out by other authors and their work is noted. The earliest reference to the problem is in 1975 and it is noted that the same applies today (McSherry 1997).

The underlying evidence from the study is that the respondents' knowledge of research is poor. The main reason behind this lack of knowledge seems to be that there was a research deficit in training. Despite this lack of knowledge, the vast majority of registered nurses do agree in principle with the concept of evidence-based practice. The author feels this may be an indication of the pressure many nurses find themselves under in ensuring that their clinical practice is based on evidence. Nurses take their responsibility of providing evidence-based care seriously and as such see the need to critically evaluate literature to aid the delivery of that care. What appears to be the case is that the skills to perform critical evaluation and to basically understand the research process are lacking (Cleverly 1998).

Conclusion

The conclusion is fully supported by the research findings and the implications of the study are identified. Again, the use of key literature adds impetus to the text and the importance and rationale behind the study is always evident. The limitations are fully expressed which makes it possible to put the findings into even greater context.

Recommendations

The recommendations apply only to the hospital population where the research took place. (This was previously explained by the author in assessing the limitations of the study.) They do, however, seem to echo the recommendations which have spanned several decades (Abdellah 1969 and Mullhall 1997). Many of the recommendations are relevant to many nurses and will probably offer an amount of scientific backing in a situation that they may have been aware of or suspected.

Relevance of the study to the nursing profession and particularly my own area of nursing practice

Traditionally, nursing has been led by institutional policies and politics, and has been carried out with an intuitive, trial and error practice. As a result of this, nurses are second-class citizens and are viewed by other professions and the public as in an ancillary occupation (Fawcett 1980). Virtue has always been at the heart of nurse education and it is widely characterised by the inclusion of moral values and virtues rather than intellectual prowess. This has resulted in the slow development of an intellectual self-confident culture in nursing (Rafferty 1996). One way forward is to enlarge the knowledge needed by scientific research and it is therefore the duty of nurses to conduct investigations of nursing phenomena (Fawcett 1980). According to Maloney (1992), since 1970 nurses have begun to value research more than in previous decades, and, as nursing moves more towards full professional status, it creates its research productivity. It is, however, acknowledged that the youthfulness of nursing as a professional body is illustrated in its limited quantity of research generated knowledge on which to base practice (Glasper 1997). Despite this, nurses are expected to make the move towards professionalism and utilise research to provide care that is evidence-based (Castledine 1997a). The author of the study feels this is an unrealistic goal if education falls short of equipping nurses with the adequate skills to evaluate and undertake research. Fawcett (1980) argued that it was the nurse's duty to become research aware and suggested that nursing practice not based upon research is unethical.

Research in any field has always been attributed an aura of mystique and authority, and the profession of nursing is no exception. This is due to its irrelevance to everyday nursing practice and it is often perceived as an elite activity and admired for its intellecturalism (Mulhall 1997). This, it has been suggested, has led to a hegemonic culture of research, and that hegemonic processes are at work within research (Mulhall 1995a, cited in Mulhall 1997). The subordinated population (nurses in general) have little chance of gaining experience in the research process as they are denied the experience of grappling with the problems of actually doing research. They are also denied the experience of 'living' the culture of the researcher but, at the same time, they are expected to utilise the findings of research (Mulhall 1997).

There are, as indicated above, plenty of obstacles in the way of nurses who wish to gain an insight into research. However, Hicks (1997) feels that nurses may have a psychological resistance, and that one possible reason for undermining nursing research is its relative newness. What is alarming is that the excuse of newness has been used for many years and perhaps if research had been incorporated into nurse training many years ago, nurses in general would be more at ease with the research process and the evaluation of research papers.

The author's recommendations take all the above into account and are relevant to all nurses largely because nurses' responsibilities are fundamentally the same and research and educational needs are similar regardless of grade. The author basically recommends facilities that can offer nurses of all grades the opportunity to gain support, to discuss finding and to obtain relevant guidance and information. Many of these recommendations are already available to local practice nurses in the form of practice nurse forums (support and dissemination of research) and good quality research education which is funded by The Trent Focus Group. The General Practice Research Framework (GPRF), which was established in 1973, gives members of the primary care team the opportunity to take part in research and practice nurses can be key players (Martin 1997). It is beneficial to the individual nurses taking part in the research because we learn how to do research if we actually take part in it (Bell 1996).

The conclusions of the study are relevant to the area of practice nursing and the study has highlighted areas of concern as a consequence. Practice nursing involves many duties which are deemed part of the 'extended role', and evidence-based care and the extended role of the nurse are infinitely linked. The philosophy of caring and research, on the other hand, are incongruous (Glasper 1997).

Role extension is linked with technological advances in medicine and role expansion appears to be more likely to succeed in community health orientated services (Hugh and Wainwright 1994). Nurses need to be aware of major studies to keep themselves up-to-date, and should also be aware of complaints and litigation trends in their speciality (Tingle 1997). Evidence-based practice is also linked with cost effectiveness in the NHS, but not all nursing problems are capable of being reduced to clear issues that can be solved by scientific needs. Many of the problems also require artistry to find a solution (White 1997).

Nurses need to have good objective skills, they need to be purposeful, reflective and questioning, and with this in mind, evidence-based nursing should always maintain a balance between research on a clinical subject and information that has been gained from the patient. There is no substitute for nurses' clinical judgement based on what a patient has to say (Castledine 1997b).

In conclusion, the study was deemed a highly credible and interesting piece of research which has stimulated further reading to gain a more in-depth insight into the research question. The conclusions and recommendations of the study are largely transferable to the area of practice nursing but also to nursing in general. The author, by looking at nurses' knowledge of research and their attitudes and feelings about it, has revealed that a fundamental 'gap' exists in nurse education, which, left unquestioned, will be detrimental to the profession of nursing. Essentially, nursing research is about patients and providing the best quality care for them (Watson 1998). Research should not be assessed in terms of a payoff for nursing rather than promise for the nursing profession (Dickoff 1975). Nurses do need to take an interest in research *per se* because if nurses do not contribute to the wider research and development agenda, they cannot make a contribution at the patient care level (McKenna 1998).

References

Abdellah, F. (1969) The nature of nursing science, *Nursing Research* 18, 390–8.

Ackerman, B. and Lyons, R. (1981) *Research Methods for Nurses*. New York, McGraw Hill.

Bell, J. (1996) *Doing Your Research Project, A Guide for the First-Time Researcher in Education and Social Science*, 2nd edn Buckingham, Open University Press.

Burns, N. and Grove, S. (1993) *The Practice of Nursing Research: Conduct, Critique and Utilisation* London, Saunders.

Castledine, G. (1997a) Assessing the future of nursing research, *British Journal of Nursing* 6, 3, 179.

Castledine, G. (1997b) Evidence-based nursing: Where is the evidence? *British Journal of Nursing* 6, 5.

Clark, E. (1994) *Research Awareness, Module 10, Evaluating Research* London, Distance Learning Centre, South Bank University.

Cleverly, D. (1998) Nursing research – taking an active interest, *Nurse Education Today* 18, 267–72.

Clifford, C. and Gough, S. (1990) *Nursing Research* New York, Prentice Hall.

Cormack, D.F.S. (1996) *The Research Process in Nursing* Oxford, Blackwell Scientific Publications.

Coyne, I.T. (1997) Sampling in qualitative research. Purposeful and theoretical sampling: merging or clear boundaries? *Journal of Advanced Nursing* 26, 623–30.

Department of Health (1989) *Working for Patients* London, HMSO.

Department of Health (1992) *The Patients' Charter: Raising the Standard* London, HMSO.

Department of Health (1993a) *Research for Health* London, DoH.

Department of Health (1993b) *Report of the Taskforce on the Strategy for Research in Nursing, Midwifery and Health Visiting* London, DoH.

Department of Health (1997) *The New NHS Modern, Dependable* London, DoH.

Dickoff, J., James, P. and Semradek, J. (1975) Research Part 1: A stance for nursing research-tenacity or inquiry, *Nursing Research* 24, 2, 84–8.

Dyson, J. (1996) Research: Promoting positive attitudes through education, *Journal of Advanced Nursing* 26, 608–12.

Fawcett, J. (1980) A declaration of nursing independence: The relation of theory and research to nursing practice, *Journal of Nursing Administration* 10, 36–9.

Funk, G.S., Champagn, M.T., Wiese, R.A. and Tornquist, E.M. (1993) Barriers: The barriers to Research Utilisation Scale, *Clinical Methods* 39–45. Cited in McSherry R. (1997) What do registered nurses and midwives feel and know about research, *Journal of Advanced Nursing*, 225, 985–98.

Glasper, E.A. (1997) Is the quest for evidence-based care detrimental to children's nursing? *British Journal of Nursing* 6, 21, 1253–5.

Hawthorne, P.J. (1983) Principles of research: A checklist, *Nursing Times* Aug 31.

Hek, G. (1995), Methods of collecting data, *Journal of Community Nursing* May 1995, 4–8.

Hek, G. (1996) Critical evaluation, *Journal of Community Nursing* 10, 6, 4–6.

Hicks, C. (1990) *Research and Statistics* New York, Prentice Hall.

Hicks, C. (1997) The dilemma of incorporating research into clinical practice, *British Journal of Nursing* 6, 9, 511–15.

Hunt, G. and Wainwright, P. (eds) (1994) *Expanding the Role of the Nurse* Oxford, Blackwell Scientific Publications.

Leighton-Beck, L. (1997) Networking: Putting research at the heart of professional practice, *British Journal of Nursing* 6, 2, 120–2.

McKenna, H. (1998) Nursing and the wider R&D agenda: Influence and contribution *NT Research* 3, 2.

McSherry, R. (1997) What do nurses and midwives feel and know about research? *Journal of Advanced Nursing* 25, 985–98.

Maloney, M.M. (1992) *Professionalization of Nursing Current Issues and Trends*, 2nd edn Philadelphia, J.B. Lippincott Company.

Martin J. (1997) Research network for general practice, *Practice Nurse* 14, 6, 372–6.

Mulhall, A. (1995a) *Research: Evaluation and Utilisation. Study Guide*, London, Distance Learning Centre, Southbank University. Cited in Mulhall A. (1997) Nursing research: Our world not theirs? *Journal of Advanced Nursing* 25, 969–6.

Ogier, M. (1992) *Reading Research* London, Scutari Press.

Polit, D. and Hungler, B. (1991), *Nursing Research* New York, J.B. Lippincott.

Rafferty, A.M. (1996) *Politics of Nursing Knowledge*, London, Routledge.

Stokes, J.E. (1981) Utilisation of research findings. In Krampitzi, S.D. and Paviovich, N. (eds) *Reading for Nursing Research* St Louis, Mosby,

227–34. Cited in McSherry R. (1997) What do nurses and midwives feel and know about research? *Journal of Advanced Nursing* 25, 985–98.

Tingle, J. (1997) Legal problems in the operating theatre: Learning from mistakes, *British Journal of Nursing* 6, 15.

United Kingdom Central Council for Nurses, Midwives and Health Visitors (1992b) *The Scope of Professional Practice* London, UKCC.

Watson, D. (1998) Developing the capacity of nursing and midwifery research: The view from higher education, *NT Research* 3, 2, 93–9.

White, S.J. (1997) Evidence-based practice and nursing: The new panacea? *British Journal of Nursing* 6, 3.

Index